Healing
Fatty
Liver
Disease

Healing
Fatty
Liver
Disease

A Complete Health & Diet Guide
Including 100 Recipes

Dr. Maitreyi Raman, MD, MSc, FRCPC,
Angela Sirounis, BSc, RD, **&**
Jennifer Shrubsole, BSc, RD

Robert
ROSE

For complete cataloguing information, see page 273.

Disclaimer
This book is a general guide only and should never be a substitute for the skill, knowledge, and experience of
a qualified medical professional dealing with the facts, circumstances, and symptoms of a particular case.

The nutritional, medical, and health information presented in this book is based on the research, training,
and professional experience of the authors, and is true and complete to the best of their knowledge. However,
this book is intended only as an informative guide for those wishing to know more about health, nutrition,
and medicine; it is not intended to replace or countermand the advice given by the reader's personal
physician. Because each person and situation is unique, the author and the publisher urge the reader to
check with a qualified health-care professional before using any procedure where there is a question as to
its appropriateness. A physician should be consulted before beginning any exercise program. The author
and the publisher are not responsible for any adverse effects or consequences resulting from the use of the
information in this book. It is the responsibility of the reader to consult a physician or other qualified health-
care professional regarding his or her personal care.

This book contains references to products that may not be available everywhere. The intent of the
information provided is to be helpful; however, there is no guarantee of results associated with the
information provided. Use of brand names is for educational purposes only and does not imply endorsement.

The recipes in this book have been carefully tested by our kitchen and our tasters. To the best of our
knowledge, they are safe and nutritious for ordinary use and users. For those people with food or other
allergies, or who have special food requirements or health issues, please read the suggested contents of each
recipe carefully and determine whether or not they may create a problem for you. All recipes are used at the
risk of the consumer. We cannot be responsible for any hazards, loss, or damage that may occur as a result of
any recipe use. For those with special needs, allergies, requirements, or health problems, in the event of any
doubt, please contact your medical adviser prior to the use of any recipe.

Design and Production: Kevin Cockburn/PageWave Graphics Inc.
Editors: Bob Hilderley, Senior Editor, Health; and Sue Sumeraj, Recipes
Copyeditor: Kelly Jones
Proofreader: Sheila Wawanash
Indexer: Gillian Watts
Illustrations: Kveta/Three in a Box
Cover Photos: Colin Erricson

Cover images (*from left to right*): Tandoori Haddock (page 219), Italian Seafood Stew (page 224) and
    Vegetable Quinoa Salad (page 194)

We acknowledge the financial support of the Government of Canada through the Book Publishing Industry
Development Program (BPIDP) for our publishing activities.

Published by Robert Rose Inc.
120 Eglinton Avenue East, Suite 800, Toronto, Ontario, Canada M4P 1E2
Tel: (416) 322-6552 Fax: (416) 322-6936
www.robertrose.ca

Printed and bound in Canada

1 2 3 4 5 6 7 8 9 FP 21 20 19 18 17 16 15 14 13

Contents

Introduction

Surprisingly, the most common liver disease seen in the developed world is not viral hepatitis or cirrhosis of the liver but rather fatty liver disease, specifically nonalcoholic fatty liver disease (NAFLD).

Surprisingly, the most common liver disease seen in the developed world is not viral hepatitis or cirrhosis of the liver but rather fatty liver disease, specifically nonalcoholic fatty liver disease (NAFLD). Even though there are many types of liver disease, NAFLD is perhaps the least recognized! Most people discover they have fatty liver disease during tests for other common conditions, such as heart disease or diabetes. When discovered, fatty liver disease might have progressed to hepatitis, fibrosis, and cirrhosis. Cirrhosis cannot be reversed and results in death unless a donor liver can be found and transplanted successfully.

This disconnection between the most common cause of liver disease and its underwhelming recognition is difficult to fathom. The lack of understanding is clearly dangerous, but it is not easy to overcome, because few obvious symptoms accompany this condition. In fact, in the early phases of this disease, there are almost no symptoms. The symptoms that may be present with NAFLD are often nonspecific (meaning that they can be seen with other conditions) and may be dismissed as not sufficiently relevant or clinically meaningful to warrant further investigations. Once the common symptoms typically associated with liver disease are present, it usually signifies that the disease has progressed to an advanced stage. Prognosis is guarded.

Good management of NAFLD can best be facilitated through a multidisciplinary, holistic approach in conjunction with a registered dietitian, gastroenterologist/ hepatologist, exercise therapist, and psychologist.

Diagnosis is typically determined by tests conducted by a gastroenterologist (digestive-system specialist) or hepatologist (liver specialist). Many health-care professionals are learning how to manage this condition with lifestyle changes, behavioral modification, medications, and dietary therapy, but there are still some physicians who may not be entirely familiar with this condition. Good management of NAFLD can best be facilitated through a multidisciplinary, holistic approach in conjunction with a registered dietitian, gastroenterologist/ hepatologist, exercise therapist, and psychologist. We have assembled such a group to contribute to this book. A multidisciplinary approach offers the greatest chance of long-term success. Management strategies include alcohol abstinence, prescription medications, nutritional supplements, physical exercise, and dietary therapy, which is the focus of this book. The diet program recommended in this book includes therapeutic food choices, convenient menu plans, and recipes that help manage and, in most cases, reverse fatty liver disease.

Despite the high prevalence of NAFLD, very few books have been written on this topic. I found this odd because numerous patients in my clinical practice persistently request a good resource of information for understanding and managing their condition. This book will provide you with the best information available today about your liver disease and the factors that predispose you toward NAFLD, management strategies targeted at achieving weight loss and obtaining better control over diabetes, and a complete dietary guide that includes a series of recipes to assist you on this journey. These strategies are evidence-based and are founded on the most recent research published in the best-known medical journals. The recipes have been tested in our kitchen, and each recipe includes a nutritional analysis to assist you in making sure your meals are well-balanced among the food groups.

Meaningful gains can be made with this book as a practical guide to get your liver into better shape and to avoid the dreaded complications of advanced liver disease, notably cirrhosis of the liver. By implementing these suggested strategies early, you can reverse any detrimental changes in the liver that are already present. If you suspect you may have nonalcoholic fatty liver disease, please don't delay. See your doctor and consider adopting the management strategies we describe in *Healing Fatty Liver Disease*.

> Despite the high prevalence of NAFLD, very few books have been written on this topic.

Case Histories

Case histories reveal the challenges and triumphs you can experience as a patient with fatty liver disease. You will no doubt see yourself in many of the cases presented in this book. Learn from other patients — and watch your health return.

Case History

Robert Greene

Robert is 41 years old and recently applied for life insurance. He got a surprising letter from the life insurance company rejecting his application due to liver blood tests that were found to be higher than normal. He was quite concerned by this finding and went to his family physician for more information regarding what might be causing this problem. His doctor thought that he might be drinking too much alcohol, which is a common reason for high liver tests, or he had hepatitis.

Robert was shocked at the thought of hepatitis. He was concerned that he might have hepatitis and was going to suffer serious consequences. He could not think of any specific reason why he might have hepatitis. Whenever Robert had heard the term "hepatitis" used in the past, it was in the context of a liver infection that was contracted during a trip to Mexico, or somewhere sunny and warm. In fact, he remembered those television commercials about hepatitis quite well, and saw something about being vaccinated for hepatitis before traveling. Unfortunately, Robert never did get vaccinated and traveled to Cuba just last summer. His family doctor asked him about risk factors for hepatitis, such as unprotected sex or using intravenous drugs. He did admit to having unprotected sex, though not in Cuba.

Now he was feeling increasingly anxious about his blood tests and wanted more information regarding the next steps in diagnosis. Robert's doctor conducted a detailed physical examination and sent him for an ultrasound imaging study. He changed the diagnosis from hepatitis to nonalcoholic fatty liver disease (NAFLD) and sat down with Robert to discuss ways of managing this disease.

Mary Smith

Mary Smith is a 43-year-old housewife and mother of three children under the age of 10. Although she was lean during childhood and young adulthood, she has been unable to lose the weight gained during her pregnancies. She currently is 200 pounds. Her life has been consumed by her children in recent years. Monday and Wednesday afternoons find Mary shuttling her children to piano lessons followed by figure skating. Tuesday and Thursday evenings involve driving her children to soccer practice. Her neighborhood does not support a school bus system, necessitating school drop-offs and pick-ups. Over the past 10 years, Mary has steadily gained weight. Her physical activity has dwindled and her energy is quite poor. She is constantly fatigued.

Recently, Mary has had a vague discomfort located under her right rib cage. At first she thought she might have injured herself while shoveling the driveway, but this pain has been persistent for more than 2 months. Mary finally went to her family doctor, who sent her for an ultrasound of the abdomen. The ultrasound showed diffuse fatty infiltration of the liver, known as nonalcoholic fatty liver disease. The pain below the right rib cage that Mary was feeling is another symptom of this common condition. There are many causes for abdominal pain, including gallstones, inflammation of the pancreas, blocked intestine, appendicitis, and irritable bowel syndrome. Mary's medical history, a physical examination, an ultrasound, and further blood work confirmed that she had nonalcoholic fatty liver disease (NAFLD). For Mary, the first step in managing this disease was to lose weight. Being overweight or obese has become the chief cause of fatty liver disease once overuse of alcohol is ruled out.

Most cases are much more complex than the ones presented here. In compiling a case, we aim to address the predominant condition, but we also hope to identify sub-clinical health concerns that may be contributing to less than perfect health. These cases are composites, based on several individual cases from our medical and nutritional counseling practices.

Part 1
Understanding Fatty Liver Disease

CHAPTER 1

What Is Fatty Liver Disease?

Case History

Tina White

Tina is a 45-year-old high school science teacher. She recently had some routine blood tests done as part of her annual check-up. The tests indicated she had problems with her liver, and her doctor referred her for an ultrasound, which revealed she had fat in her liver, technically known as nonalcoholic fatty liver disease. She had never heard of this before. The only liver diseases she knew about were jaundice in children, hepatitis from unprotected sex, and cirrhosis of the liver from drinking excessive amounts of alcohol. But she had never experienced jaundice, nor had she had unprotected sex. She didn't even drink alcohol! When she met with her doctor she asked to know more about this nonalcoholic fatty liver disease, which her doctor abbreviated as NAFLD. What is NAFLD? What are the symptoms? What causes this disease? What are the outcomes? Can I die from this condition? What can I do to "cure" this disease? Tina set out to find more information so she could better understand and manage this disease ...

(continued on page 19)

Liver Basics

Fatty liver disease is not a high-profile medical condition and is certainly not well-known, but approximately one-third of the North American population has fatty liver disease, and 5% to 10% of these cases will progress from a benign state to cirrhosis of the liver. Cirrhosis cannot be reversed and results in death. Clearly, there is a need to understand the basics of fatty liver disease, which can be reversed before progressing to cirrhosis.

Prevalence and Incidence
- Nonalcoholic fatty liver disease (NAFLD) is the most common cause of liver disease in North America.
- In the United States and Canada, 30% of the population has NAFLD. That is almost one in three people!
- Within the United States, there is a surprisingly varied prevalence of NAFLD based on ethnicity: 45% of Hispanics,

33% of Caucasians, and 24% of African-Americans are affected by NAFLD.

- The incidence of NAFLD is associated with the rising incidence of obesity and diabetes in the Western world.

FAQ

Q. Does nonalcoholic fatty liver disease affect children?

A. NAFLD is not unique to adults and has been reported in children as young as 2 years of age, although this is quite rare. However, NAFLD is being identified with greater frequency in older children and teenagers. It is estimated that 1 in 10 Canadian child is overweight. This number has tripled in the last decade. NAFLD affects 3% of all children, and more than 50% of obese children.

Liver Disease Spectrum

NAFLD does not consist of one single type of liver abnormality. It is a broad term used to describe various findings in the liver that range in severity from mild disease at one end of the spectrum to severe disease at the other end.

In NAFLD, there is a buildup of fat droplets in the liver tissue. Normally, fat should only live in fat cells. When fat starts to accumulate in greater quantities in organs where fat would not usually reside, this is a sign that these organs, such as the liver, are being negatively impacted by the presence of fat.

When fat is present in the liver and there are no other findings that suggest a more advanced disease, this is called simple steatosis, or simple liver fat. When findings suggest the presence of simple liver fat with associated inflammation and scarring, it is called nonalcoholic steatohepatitis (NASH).

NAFLD or NASH?

Often the distinction between simple liver fat and liver fat plus inflammation or scarring can only be made using invasive tools, such as a liver biopsy. The distinction between simple steatosis and NASH is often necessary to determine because we know that simple steatosis usually carries a benign prognosis and does not result in serious liver-related consequences. In contrast, NASH is a progressive abnormality, meaning that people with NASH may progress with greater frequency to the more ominous consequences of cirrhosis and advanced liver disease. Approximately 20% of patients with NASH will develop cirrhosis. If your doctor has determined you have NASH, you must work hard to make lifestyle changes that reduce your risk of developing cirrhosis of the liver.

Liver Disease Spectrum

Nonalcoholic Fatty Liver Disease

Nonalcoholic fatty liver disease (NAFLD)

Simple steatosis

Fat in liver tissue

Nonalcoholic steatohepatitis (NASH)

Steatohepatitis

Fat in liver tissue + inflammation and scarring

Alcoholic-Related Liver Disease

Simple steatosis

Steatohepatitis

Liver Disease Progression

Healthy Liver

Fatty Liver
Fat deposits in liver tissue
Enlargement of the liver

Hepatitis
Inflammation
Fibrosis
Scar tissue
Liver cell injury

Cirrhosis
Scar tissue hardens
Liver failure
Death

FAQ

Q. **What is the difference between nonalcoholic and alcoholic fatty liver disease?**

A. Alcohol consumption can result in simple steatosis (fatty liver) or steatohepatitis (fatty liver plus inflammation and scarring). In fact, if you look under the microscope at liver samples from patients with fatty liver disease and patients who drink excess alcohol, their livers will appear identical.

Alcoholic liver disease usually occurs after years of drinking too much alcohol. The duration of alcohol consumption and the amount of alcohol consumed typically determine the likelihood of developing liver disease and the severity. Alcohol consumption may cause swelling and inflammation, otherwise known as hepatitis, in the liver. Over time, this can lead to scarring of the liver, fibrosis, and eventually cirrhosis of the liver.

In this respect, alcoholic liver disease is identical to nonalcoholic fatty liver disease. It is not possible to differentiate between the two by looking at blood tests, or even liver biopsy, because the two disease conditions are almost identical. The diagnosis of alcoholic versus nonalcoholic fatty liver disease is determined purely through a detailed and accurate evaluation of a patient's history of alcohol use. The early stages of alcoholic liver disease characterized by fatty liver or hepatitis are almost completely reversible with abstinence.

Tough Terms

The language of liver disease can be confusing. To simplify terminology without sacrificing precision, we will use the following terms:

- Steatosis, nonalcoholic fatty liver disease (NAFLD), and fatty liver disease will be used interchangeably, with fatty liver disease favored for its simplicity. Fatty liver disease is the focus of this book.
- Steatohepatitis (fat plus inflammation and scarring) will be used interchangeably with nonalcoholic steatohepatitis (NASH).
- When we are dealing with alcohol-influenced steatosis and steatohepatitis, we will refer to these conditions simply as alcoholic-related liver disease as a counterpart to nonalcoholic fatty liver disease.

DID YOU KNOW?

Gender Difference

Alcohol affects men and women very differently. Women may consume much smaller amounts of alcohol than men and yet suffer the same adverse consequences as men who drink far greater quantities of alcohol.

Anatomy of the Liver

Understanding fatty liver disease begins by learning how the liver works, specifically the anatomy and pathophysiology of this organ. The liver is a complex organ and is involved in a wide variety of interactions with other organs and systems, making it vulnerable to dysfunction.

Anatomy of the Abdomen

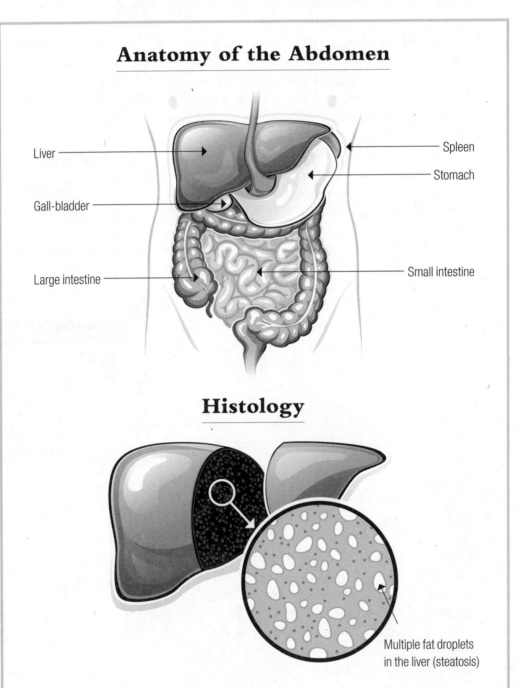

Liver

Spleen

Stomach

Gall-bladder

Large intestine

Small intestine

Histology

Multiple fat droplets in the liver (steatosis)

The liver is the largest organ in the body. It weighs between 3 and 3.5 pounds (1.44 and 1.66 kg). The liver is located behind the ribs in the right upper portion of the abdomen. It is shaped like a triangle. It has two large sections, called the right and left lobes, and consists of many bile ducts, blood vessels, and specialized cells. The gallbladder sits under the liver, along with parts of the pancreas and intestines.

Functions of the Liver

The liver's main function is to filter the blood coming from the digestive tract before it passes through to the rest of the body. Other functions of the liver include:

- Clearing or detoxifying the body of waste products, drugs, and other poisonous substances
- Producing proteins to clot blood and stop excessive bleeding
- Producing immune factors that help remove bacteria from the bloodstream to fight infection
- Releasing bile, which is a substance that helps digest food and absorb nutrients

Any disruption of these functions can cause liver disease. Liver diseases are suspected when common symptoms are detected, risk factors for liver disease are present, and abnormal liver conditions are assessed through blood tests.

Signs and Symptoms

Most people with fatty liver disease do not have symptoms. This is the scary part. It is a little like having high blood pressure — the majority of people with high blood pressure are walking around with it but have no idea they are affected. Sometimes, high blood pressure comes to light, and fatty liver disease is officially diagnosed only when these patients present with another serious complication, such as a heart attack or stroke.

Right Upper Quadrant Pain

Although symptoms of NAFLD are not common, if present, the most common symptom is pain just below the right rib cage. This is termed right upper quadrant (RUQ) pain. This pain is usually described as a dull, steady pain present throughout the day. It is seldom made better or worse by eating. It is rarely so debilitating that it interferes with daily activities.

Most people who suffer from this discomfort acknowledge that this pain exists, but they rarely suffer greatly from it.

Fatigue and Exhaustion

Additional symptoms of fatty liver disease include fatigue and exhaustion, which are strongly associated with obesity. The cycle of existing fatigue in NAFLD often precludes the desire to engage in physical activity, often prohibiting successful treatment of the disease. Contrary to popular belief, however, exercise in the context of obesity stimulates hormones that will raise energy levels and affect mood quite favorably, with a positive benefit for treating fatty liver disease.

Associated Symptoms

Other symptoms that are associated with liver disease are typically not seen in NAFLD unless the disease has advanced to the point of cirrhosis or severe scarring of the liver, precluding normal function of the liver.

Jaundice

Jaundice (yellowing of the skin and eyes) is not likely related to NAFLD, but in a very advanced form of NAFLD, jaundice warrants further evaluation for the presence of these symptoms.

Edema (Swelling of the Ankles)

Similarly, persistent swelling of the ankles from fluid retention and increasing abdominal girth from fluid rather than fat are seen only in advanced cases of liver disease, not with routine NAFLD. If these symptoms are present, further assessment for other causes of these symptoms should be undertaken.

Cirrhosis

If you have been diagnosed with cirrhosis of the liver from NAFLD, it is imperative to monitor symptoms diligently, because development of any of the following symptoms could signify a failing liver:

- Swelling in the ankles or legs
- Swelling in the belly from fluid
- Confusion, forgetfulness, or memory impairment
- Passing blood with bowel movements
- Passing black, tarry stools
- Vomiting blood

Ruling Out Concomitant Conditions

Despite the increased frequency of fatty liver disease in a person with these symptoms, it is still quite possible that other disease states (ones that cause liver abnormalities) may still be present. Although the diagnosis of NAFLD may be suspected based on these clinical characteristics, further tests need to be performed to rule out concomitant liver conditions, something that is essential to be done, especially if the laboratory liver tests are inconsistent or abnormal.

Case History (continued)

Tina

Tina was assessed by her liver specialist, who sent her for a number of tests. The tests confirmed the diagnosis of NAFLD. She was told that her weight gain during the past 10 years, her sedentary lifestyle, and her high cholesterol level all predisposed her toward NAFLD. Tina did not drink any alcohol. Her liver specialist suggested a liver biopsy to determine whether Tina had simple steatosis or NASH. Tina decided to wait on making that decision until she was more informed about the risks and benefits of doing so.

CHAPTER 2

How Is Fatty Liver Disease Diagnosed?

Case History

Mark Jones

Mark is 50 years old. He recently retired following a successful career in finance. His busy professional life entailed traveling internationally for business and wining and dining high-powered clients, leaving virtually no time to care for himself. Mark recently had an ultrasound of his abdomen because of discomfort in the middle part of his belly. His ultrasound was normal, but the report did mention a concern about fatty liver disease. The family doctor sent Mark for further blood tests, including a check of his liver enzymes. The liver enzymes were found to be twice the upper limit of normal. When Mark asked his family doctor what this finding meant, the doctor told Mark that he had NAFLD, but that with some weight loss, the fat content in his liver should improve. Nonetheless, Mark was referred to a liver specialist.

When the liver specialist assessed Mark 2 months later, and a complete panel of blood tests was performed, Mark was diagnosed with hepatitis C. He was absolutely shocked at this news. Mark wanted more information about this disease and wondered why NAFLD had been the original diagnosis ...

(continued on page 27)

The onset of NAFLD can be suspected either from your medical history or by physical examination. During a regular physical examination or evaluation of a routine blood test, your doctor may suspect a liver problem, which he will follow up with further examination, blood tests, imaging studies, and , if necessary, biopsy to confirm a diagnosis. Once this suspicion is raised, it needs to be confirmed. Diagnosis is by exclusion as other similar conditions are ruled out.

Diagnostic Tests for NAFLD

- Physical examination
- Blood tests (including liver enzyme levels)
- Imaging studies
- Biopsy

Physical Examination

In routine NAFLD, when you have a physical examination, your doctor might not find anything abnormal. Although no one symptom or sign positively indicates fatty liver disease, the following conditions may be sufficient to prompt your doctor to request blood tests and imaging studies to help consolidate a diagnosis:

- *High blood pressure*: Elevated blood pressure may be a clue pointing toward NAFLD; however, high blood pressure is so common that it may mean nothing at all.
- *RUQ pain*: Similarly, when your doctor examines your abdomen, you may feel some tenderness or discomfort in the right upper abdomen. Again, this discomfort may be present for any number of reasons and does not mean that you have NAFLD.
- *Enlarged liver*: Sometimes, a routine physical exam may reveal a large liver. If this is the case, then this finding would need to be confirmed by further testing with imaging modalities, such as an ultrasound. A large liver may be seen in NAFLD, but it may also be seen in other conditions.
- *Enlarged spleen*: A large spleen may occur in the context of NAFLD if the disease is advanced, with scarring or cirrhosis, but it may be seen in other disease states as well. A large spleen will rarely be felt.
- *Body measure*: Perhaps the most compelling or useful features pointing toward the presence of NAFLD on physical examination are height, weight and waist circumference. The probability that you have NAFLD increases with greater weight and waist circumference. Couple this with high blood pressure, and the diagnosis of NAFLD increases in likelihood tremendously.

Rule Out Alcohol

Your family doctor will try to assess your consumption of alcohol as one of the first steps in the diagnostic process. Excess alcohol consumption can result in exactly the same type of clinical picture as NAFLD. Keep in mind that the expansion for NAFLD is nonalcoholic fatty liver disease. This means that the diagnosis of NAFLD can only be provided in a setting where alcohol intake is minimal.

Possible Signs of Fatty Liver Disease
- High blood pressure
- RUQ tenderness
- Enlarged liver
- Body measure

DID YOU KNOW?

Diagnostic Criteria

In order to meet the diagnostic criteria for NAFLD, men cannot exceed two standard alcoholic beverages daily, and women cannot exceed one alcoholic beverage daily. If alcohol consumption is greater than these specified amounts, we are not dealing with NAFLD — but may be dealing with alcoholic-related liver disease. This is certainly a cause for fat deposits in the liver, but alcoholic-related liver disease is managed quite differently.

There are differences in the allowable intake of alcohol between the sexes. Men generally metabolize alcohol more efficiently than women. Therefore, they can drink slightly more alcohol than women without sustaining ill health effects as a consequence.

Incidental Abnormal Blood Tests

Fatty liver disease is most commonly diagnosed through incidental abnormal blood work. Typically, your family physician has sent you for blood tests for some unrelated reason, such as an annual physical examination or for blood work for insurance purposes. These types of blood tests usually screen for common conditions, including abnormal liver enzyme levels, which may suggest underlying liver disease. Higher than accepted normal ranges can cause some anxiety for the patient and prompt the family physician to undertake a complete workup to assess the cause of these abnormalities.

Blood Panel

Usually, a panel of more comprehensive blood work is then recommended by your family physician to determine the cause of these abnormal liver tests. In many cases, your physician may recommend repeating the liver tests a few months later, to assess if the abnormalities are sustained or were part of an isolated episode. In the face of persistent liver test abnormalities, your doctor will likely refer you to a gastroenterologist or liver specialist, otherwise known as a hepatologist.

Liver Enzymes

One of the most common findings in NAFLD is abnormal liver-specific blood tests. These liver-specific blood tests include the level of liver enzymes, also known as aminotransferases. The aminotransferases include alanine aminotransferase (ALT) and aspartate aminotransferase (AST). Another important liver test is the gamma glutamyl transpeptidase (GGT). An ultrasound of the abdomen is a useful complement to liver enzyme tests when determining the presence of NAFLD.

Liver enzymes are sensitive markers of liver injury or inflammation. The presence of conventional NAFLD risk factors and abnormal liver enzymes increase the probability of NAFLD. However, because there are many reasons why abnormal liver enzymes may occur, including diseases both related and not related to the liver, the presence of liver disease should not be automatically assumed if liver enzymes are abnormal. Although abnormal liver enzymes are consistent with NAFLD, they can be seen in many other liver diseases. NAFLD can occur in the presence of normal liver enzymes, and having normal liver enzymes does not automatically rule out the likelihood of having NAFLD. With NAFLD, there may be some fluctuation of the liver enzymes on a month-to-month basis.

Blood Glucose Levels

High blood glucose, otherwise known as glucose intolerance or diabetes, is a risk factor for NAFLD. In fact, NAFLD patients with diabetes tend to have more advanced disease than patients without diabetes. Patients with diabetes are more likely to have NASH (fat plus inflammation and scarring) than non-diabetic patients. Therefore, an accurate assessment regarding the presence or absence of diabetes needs to be undertaken.

Generally, a fasting blood sugar level is sufficient to make a diagnosis of diabetes; however, additional tests, such as a glucose tolerance test, are sometimes necessary. A glucose tolerance test involves consuming a sugar drink and testing for blood sugar levels in serial measurements.

Triglycerides and Cholesterol

When NAFLD is suspected, it is necessary to check levels of fasting triglycerides and cholesterol. These lipids are not only risk factors for NAFLD, they can also influence disease severity. Generally, it is recommended to not eat or drink for 12 hours prior to these tests.

Complete Blood Count

Your doctor will routinely perform these lab tests in the presence of abnormal liver enzymes or if the diagnosis of NAFLD is suspected. In advanced cases of NAFLD or in advanced cases of any liver disease (cirrhosis), the ability of the liver to function may be compromised to a greater or lesser degree. This may result in bleeding through the gastrointestinal (GI) tract, leading to low iron stores and low hemoglobin. This information will be captured in the complete blood count (CBC). If advanced scarring or cirrhosis is present, the platelet count, another component of the CBC, may be reduced. Platelets are blood cells responsible for the clotting process. Similarly, white blood cells, another component of the CBC, may be reduced. White blood cells are necessary to fight infection.

Other functions of the liver, such as the production of proteins to clot blood, may be affected, leading to a high international normalized ratio (or INR), a test that measures the time it takes for blood to clot) and increased risk of bleeding. Protein synthesis in general may also be affected, leading to low levels of albumin and bilirubin.

Blood Tests to Evaluate for Other Causes of Persistent High Liver Enzymes

There are many other causes of liver disease that may present with abnormal liver blood tests. Your family doctor or liver specialist may ask you to get some of the blood tests listed here to confirm your diagnosis.

- Hepatitis B surface antigen
- Hepatitis C antibody
- Alpha 1-antitrypsin level
- Antinuclear antibody
- Anti-smooth muscle antibody
- Anti-mitochondrial antibody
- Transferrin saturation
- Ceruloplasmin

Imaging Studies

Among the various forms of imaging studies, such as CT and MIR scans, ultrasound is most commonly used.

Ultrasound Imaging

Ultrasound is commonly used to confirm symptoms. For example, an ultrasound of the abdomen is performed almost routinely as the first step in an investigation of abdominal pain. The ultrasound may reveal fat in the liver, which can then lead to the diagnosis of fatty liver disease.

In NAFLD, the ultrasound will confirm fatty deposits in the liver. Although the ultrasound may indicate the presence of fatty liver, it does not mean that other liver diseases are not present. This is especially true in the face of high liver enzymes. Usually, the radiologist or ultrasound expert will comment on mild, moderate, or severe fat infiltration of the liver.

If there is evidence of fat plus scarring of the liver, resulting in liver dysfunction, the ultrasound will provide different findings. With cirrhosis, for example, the liver may be small, nodular, and quite irregular. If the liver is not functioning properly, there may be evidence of fluid in the abdomen, otherwise known as ascites. The spleen may be large due to abnormal pressures in the major abdominal blood vessels. If these findings are identified, then advanced liver disease should be suspected and managed accordingly.

Liver Biopsy

A liver biopsy is considered the gold standard or the best tool we have to make a diagnosis of NAFLD. There are two primary reasons why a liver biopsy may be requested:

- To confirm the correct diagnosis
- To assess the severity of the underlying disease

Liver biopsy is typically reserved for individuals who have not responded well to the recommended treatments. Many of the treatments for NAFLD are based on lifestyle changes, which can be hard to achieve and even harder to maintain. Many people are unsuccessful in meeting their targets. In this circumstance, and under circumstances where individuals have been successful with lifestyle changes but their liver tests continue to be abnormal, a liver biopsy may be useful to evaluate disease severity.

Biopsy Procedure

A liver biopsy is an invasive test. This means that a sample of the liver must be removed from the body, which will be subsequently analyzed by a pathologist under a microscope. Any invasive test carries with it a chance for complication or adverse reaction.

Ultrasound Guidance

Most liver biopsies in North America are performed under ultrasound guidance. This means that a limited ultrasound is usually performed prior to the procedure. The ultrasound will help define the best part of the liver from which to take a biopsy.

Sedation

Local freezing is usually administered prior to performing the liver biopsy. In some situations, a sedative may be provided to help you relax prior to the procedure. However, this is not routinely performed. If you want a sedative prior to the procedure, ask the radiologist prior to the test, and they may be able to consider your wish.

Aspiration

Once the freezing has been administered, a long, thin needle is inserted into the liver (to the best spot identified by the ultrasound). On average, two samples of the liver are taken.

Monitoring

The actual procedure takes only a few minutes to perform. However, you will need to be monitored for at least 3 to 4 hours after the liver biopsy to ensure that you are feeling well and that there is no adverse consequence.

Complications

Some complications of liver biopsy include bleeding, perforation of a nearby organ that was not intended to be punctured, infection, and — in very small percentages — death. Death as a complication from a liver biopsy is exceedingly rare. However, because it has occurred in the past, it certainly should be mentioned.

Biopsy Limitations

Biopsy is not a perfect gold standard and has its own limitations. There is a small risk of sampling error when the biopsy is done for the purposes of NAFLD. In NAFLD, not all of the liver is affected equally. This means that there is a risk that the liver sample obtained is not affected by NAFLD. When pathologists interpret the sample, they may think that minimal disease is present even though a larger burden of disease may be present elsewhere.

Risk and Benefit Assessment

In a small set of patients with abnormal liver tests who may not fit the traditional model for an NAFLD patient, we are left wondering whether their liver disease is really from NAFLD. For example, they may be average weight or thin, or they may be using a certain medication that may cause liver injury. In these types of situations, a liver biopsy will confirm the official diagnosis and provide information regarding the severity of liver disease. The decision of pursuing a liver biopsy in NAFLD should reflect a balance between the cost of the test, the potential risks from the biopsy, and the information obtained from the biopsy that might influence the treatment plan. We generally recommend a liver biopsy to someone who has not responded satisfactorily to the recommended treatments.

Case History (continued)

Mark

On further questioning, Mark reported that on one occasion, while traveling abroad, he shared intravenous needles. This had happened more than 25 years ago, and Mark was surprised that an incident all those years ago would only come to light now, at age 50. Mark was told that even one isolated encounter with a tainted needle would be sufficient to infect him with the hepatitis C virus. Furthermore, given his lack of attention to healthy living, Mark's weight gain and obesity along with the hepatitis C virus were responsible for his abnormal liver blood tests. Mark's liver specialist then proceeded to discuss with him treatment options for the hepatitis C virus, and he was strongly encouraged to follow a healthy lifestyle, lose weight, and exercise to reduce the risk of advanced liver disease.

CHAPTER 3

What Causes Fatty Liver Disease?

Risk Factors

Establishing a diagnosis of NAFLD is achieved by evaluating for — and then excluding — other liver diseases in the context of specific risk factors. Although fatty liver disease is most often detected incidentally through abnormal blood tests, the disease is not without risk factors that cause NAFLD or that predispose to NAFLD. These predisposing factors include obesity, elevated waist circumference, diabetes, high blood pressure, and heart disease. From the examination of risk factors for NAFLD, it becomes quite evident that fatty liver disease is tightly linked to heart disease.

Excessive Alcohol Consumption

Excessive consumption of alcohol can cause fatty liver disease and affect the function of related organs and systems. In some cases, if the disease is caught at an early stage, avoiding alcohol completely may reverse the abnormal changes seen in the liver, and the liver will heal nicely. However, once scarring and cirrhosis occur, these changes may not improve completely, but at least the disease progress will usually be limited. Once the liver starts to fail, alcohol abstinence is unlikely to impact the liver function in a favorable manner.

Generally speaking, we know that women are at risk of developing liver disease from alcohol intake if they consume more than one to two standard drinks of alcohol daily. For men, the risk of liver disease increases after drinking five to six alcoholic beverages daily for 10 to 15 years. With these levels of alcohol intake, the risk of fatty liver disease, hepatitis, fibrosis, and cirrhosis all increase dramatically.

Other organ systems are affected by excess alcohol consumption too. In particular, alcohol may affect the pancreas, leading to chronic pancreatitis, which may result in severe abdominal pain, weight loss, and malnutrition. It may also affect the brain, leading to forgetfulness and memory impairment, and the heart, leading to heart failure characterized by shortness of breath, fatigue, and swelling in the legs.

Malnutrition

Many people who drink excessively ignore proper dietary and nutritional habits and are at risk of malnutrition. They may not ingest adequate amounts of vitamins and minerals for optimal health. These protective micronutrients include vitamin E, antioxidants, adequate protein, and folate.

Overweight and Obesity

Of the many risk factors for NAFLD, the strongest predisposing factor is weight status. Body mass index (BMI) is one determinant of risk ascribed to weight. The BMI is a tool used to assess, classify, and monitor body weight changes. It is a number derived from calculations based on your height and weight. Risks for numerous medical conditions increase with an overweight status and escalate exponentially with each class of obesity.

DID YOU KNOW?

Alcoholic Fatty Liver Facts

- Drinking alcohol before or after mealtimes (instead of with food) increases the risk of developing liver disease by almost three times.
- Women are affected to a greater degree than men, primarily due to a decreased presence of the enzymes that metabolize alcohol. Therefore, larger amounts of the toxic byproducts of alcohol build up in women, conveying liver damage.
- People who drink large quantities of alcohol and also have hepatitis C infection are at increased risk of having more severe liver disease.

Body Mass Index (BMI)
Calculating BMI
BMI is calculated as follows:

International (metric) units: $\text{BMI} = \text{Weight (kg)} \div (\text{Height (m)})^2$
Imperial units: $\text{BMI} = \text{Weight (lbs)} \times 703 \div (\text{Height (in)})^2$

For example, if you weigh 120 kg and are 165 cm tall, your BMI is 44.1.

$$\text{BMI} = 120 \div (1.65 \times 1.65) = 44.1$$

Alternatively, you can use the BMI chart reproduced here and on the Internet.

BMI Classifications

BMI Category (kg÷m²)	Classification	Risk of developing health problems
< 18.5	Underweight	Increased
18.5–24.9	Normal weight	Least
25.0–29.9	Overweight	Increased
30.0–34.9	Obese class 1	High
35.0–39.9	Obese class 2	Very high
≥ 40	Obese class 3	Extremely high

Interpreting BMI
Use this scale to interpret your BMI:
Normal: 19–24.9
Overweight: 25.0–29.9
Obese: greater than or equal to 30

There are three classes of obesity:
Class 1: 30.0–34.9
Class 2: 35.0–39.9
Class 3: greater than or equal to 40

BMI Limitations
This BMI calculation is for Caucasian individuals. Calculating the BMI for Asian individuals requires adjustments because of the decreased bone mass usually found in this population.

If Caucasian definitions of overweight and obesity are applied to an Asian individual, there is a risk of underestimating the likelihood of developing metabolic conditions, such as diabetes and NAFLD.

BMI should be interpreted with some caution because it does not always provide a true measurement of risk. BMI takes into consideration height and weight. There are several body factors that contribute toward total weight. These include bone mass, muscle mass, water weight, and fat mass. Although most people have a high BMI usually as a function of increased fat, it is quite possible that individuals with significant muscle mass will have a higher BMI. People with a higher BMI due to a higher percentage of muscle mass do not have the same level of risk of obesity-related diseases as people with a higher BMI due to fat mass. The proportion of people with increased muscle mass contributing toward a higher BMI is actually quite low. Taller, more muscular men may have a higher BMI that reflects increased muscle mass. This is rarely true for the rest of us. It is seldom true for women, who generally carry less muscle mass.

Measuring Waist Circumference

Due to the imperfections associated with BMI, doctors sometimes use another measure of risk to categorize the impact of weight on health conditions. Waist circumference is measured by using a measuring tape around the torso at the height of the belly button.

- *Waist limits for women:* 34.6 inches (88 cm) or less
- *Waist limits for men:* 39.4 inches (100 cm) or less

Waist circumference beyond these limits increases the risk of developing heart disease (including heart attacks and angina chest pains), certain cancers, type 2 diabetes mellitus, high blood pressure, and nonalcoholic fatty liver disease.

It is entirely conceivable that someone could have a normal BMI using the metrics provided here, but have an elevated waist circumference — and still be at risk for heart disease, cancer, and fatty liver disease. BMI and waist circumference should be used in combination when thinking ahead to optimal management of weight status.

BODY MASS INDEX TABLE

BMI	19	20	21	22	23	24	25	26	27	28	29	30	31	32	33	34	35	36
Height (inches)	Body Weight (pounds)																	
	NORMAL						OVERWEIGHT					OBESE						
58	91	96	100	105	110	115	119	124	129	134	138	143	148	153	158	162	167	172
59	94	99	104	109	114	119	124	128	133	138	143	148	153	158	163	168	173	178
60	97	102	107	112	118	123	128	133	138	143	148	153	158	163	168	174	179	184
61	100	106	111	116	122	127	132	137	143	148	153	158	164	169	174	180	185	190
62	104	109	115	120	126	131	136	142	147	153	158	164	169	175	180	186	191	196
63	107	113	118	124	130	135	141	146	152	158	163	169	175	180	186	191	197	203
64	110	116	122	128	134	140	145	151	157	163	169	174	180	186	192	197	204	209
65	114	120	126	132	138	144	150	156	162	168	174	180	186	192	198	204	210	216
66	118	124	130	136	142	148	155	161	167	173	179	186	192	198	204	210	216	223
67	121	127	134	140	146	153	159	166	172	178	185	191	198	204	211	217	223	230
68	125	131	138	144	151	158	164	171	177	184	190	197	203	210	216	223	230	236
69	128	135	142	149	155	162	169	176	182	189	196	203	209	216	223	230	236	243
70	132	139	146	153	160	167	174	181	188	195	202	209	216	222	229	236	243	250
71	136	143	150	157	165	172	179	186	193	200	208	215	222	229	236	243	250	257
72	140	147	154	162	169	177	184	191	199	206	213	221	228	235	242	250	258	265
73	144	151	159	166	174	182	189	197	204	212	219	227	235	242	250	257	265	272
74	148	155	163	171	179	186	194	202	210	218	225	233	241	249	256	264	272	280
75	152	160	168	176	184	192	200	208	216	224	232	240	248	256	264	272	279	287
76	156	164	172	180	189	197	205	213	221	230	238	246	254	263	271	279	287	295

Source: Adapted with permission from *Clinical Guidelines on the Identification, Evaluation, and Treatment of Overweight and Obesity in Adults: The Evidence Report.*

BODY MASS INDEX TABLE

BMI	37	38	39	40	41	42	43	44	45	46	47	48	49	50	51	52	53	54
Height (inches)								**Body Weight (pounds)**										
	OBESE			EXTREME OBESITY														
58	177	181	186	191	196	201	205	210	215	220	224	229	234	239	244	248	253	258
59	183	188	193	198	203	208	212	217	222	227	232	237	242	247	252	257	262	267
60	189	194	199	204	209	215	220	225	230	235	240	245	250	255	261	266	271	276
61	195	201	206	211	217	222	227	232	238	243	248	254	259	264	269	275	280	285
62	202	207	213	218	224	229	235	240	246	251	256	262	267	273	278	284	289	295
63	208	214	220	225	231	237	242	248	254	259	265	270	278	282	287	293	299	304
64	215	221	227	232	238	244	250	256	262	267	273	279	285	291	296	302	308	314
65	222	228	234	240	246	252	258	264	270	276	282	288	294	300	306	312	318	324
66	229	235	241	247	253	260	266	272	278	284	291	297	303	309	315	322	328	334
67	236	242	249	255	261	268	274	280	287	293	299	306	312	319	325	331	338	344
68	243	249	256	262	269	276	282	289	295	302	308	315	322	328	335	341	348	354
69	250	257	263	270	277	284	291	297	304	311	318	324	331	338	345	351	358	365
70	257	264	271	278	285	292	299	306	313	320	327	334	341	348	355	362	369	376
71	265	272	279	286	293	301	308	315	322	329	338	343	351	358	365	372	379	386
72	272	279	287	294	302	309	316	324	331	338	346	353	361	368	375	383	390	397
73	280	288	295	302	310	318	325	333	340	348	355	363	371	378	386	393	401	408
74	287	295	303	311	319	326	334	342	350	358	365	373	381	389	396	404	412	420
75	295	303	311	319	327	335	343	351	359	367	375	383	391	399	407	415	423	431
76	304	312	320	328	336	344	353	361	369	377	385	394	402	410	418	426	435	443

FAQ

Q. What has caused the current obesity epidemic?

A. The early 1990s marked the beginning of the age of inactivity and obesity. Rates of overweight and obesity rose to levels never previously seen. In fact, by 2006, two-thirds of North Americans were overweight or obese! These numbers are now reflected among the majority of industrialized nations. The conveniences of industrialization and socioeconomic advancement have been marked by quick access to foods that are generally ready-made, greasy, or fried, and filled with preservatives. And easy access to a family vehicle has quickly obviated the desire to walk to and from destinations. With the presence of escalators and elevators aside most staircases, seldom are individuals motivated to walk up a flight of steps when low-impact alternatives are available. These are just a few realities of our daily existence that have come to contribute toward obesity.

Food Basics

Food consists of three macronutrients — carbohydrates, proteins, and fats — and several kinds of micronutrients, which enable digestion and the absorption of macronutrients.

- Carbohydrates consist of starchy substances (vegetables, fruits, and grains), including breads, rice, pastas, muffins, and potatoes, to name a few. They provide the body with calories, or energy.
- Proteins are large molecules that consist of smaller molecules called amino acids. Proteins are the building blocks for new muscles; they are critical to the successful repair and regeneration of muscles and other tissues in the body. Proteins may be derived from either plant-based sources or animal-based sources. Legumes, including chickpeas, kidney beans, black beans, and soy beans, to mention a few, are examples of plant sources of proteins. Examples of animal-based sources of protein include any red meats, poultry, fish, and eggs.
- Fats are the most energy-dense macronutrient. When equal amounts of protein, fat, and carbohydrate are consumed, fats will provide the most energy, otherwise known as calories. Any excessive amount of fat is stored in fatty tissue, causing weight gain and sometimes obesity.

- Micronutrients include vitamins, minerals, essential fatty acids, and amino acids. Micronutrients are available in our food, but some need to be supplemented when they become deficient in the body.

Energy Imbalance

Weight gain is caused by an imbalance between energy consumed and energy expended. If you eat more macronutrients than your body requires for daily activity, you will most likely gain weight. Generally speaking, excess carbohydrate and fat consumptions are the contributing culprits toward weight gain.

Muscle Mass

Muscle mass is perhaps the key determinant of energy required. Unfortunately, muscle mass declines with age, with a greater percentage of muscle mass lost after the age of 40. Unless an active effort is applied toward maintaining and building lean muscle mass, a decline in muscle mass is inevitable. A 25-year-old active male will require more calories to carry out his usual functions than a 50-year-old active man or woman. Similarly, a 38-year-old active male construction worker will require more calories than a 38-year-old sedentary male truck driver.

Often, patients will tell me that they have no idea how the pounds have accumulated over the years. They may have been lean through their 20s and 30s, and now, in their late 40s and 50s, they find themselves 20 or 30 pounds (9 or 14 kg) heavier, despite not changing their portion sizes or quality of food eaten. I generally respond to these comments by reminding people of the fact that energy requirements are largely driven by muscle mass, and that with declining physical activity and no active attempt to build muscle mass, even previous routine portion sizes will result in fat accumulation.

With age, it becomes imperative that portion sizes and overall calorie intake are reduced — unless physical activity is increased. In the absence of a habitual culture of physical activity, one that has been created from childhood or youth, it becomes increasingly difficult to develop exercise habits in middle age, though it's not impossible with some goal and priority setting.

DID YOU KNOW?

Calorie Counting

A calorie is defined as a measure of energy. Healthy intake of calories for the average woman is about 2000 calories, and for the average man it is about 2200 calories. It takes 3500 excess calories to result in 1 pound (500 g) of weight gain. Energy requirements are based on a number of factors, including height, weight, sex, and level of activity. Exceeding the energy requirements will result in weight gain.

Macronutrient Table

Macronutrient	Calories per gram Consumed
Carbohydrate	4 kcal/g
Protein	4 kcal/g
Fat	9 kcal/g

Vegetable Sources of Protein

Protein Source	Grams of Protein per serving
Seaweed (spirulina), 1 cup (250 mL)	64
Parsley, 1 cup (250 mL)	31
Lentils, cooked, 1 cup (250 mL)	18
Black beans, cooked, 1 cup (250 mL)	15
Tofu, 3.4 oz (100 g)	20
Quinoa, cooked, 1 cup (250 mL)	9
Peanut butter, 2 tbsp (30 mL)	8
Almonds, $\frac{1}{4}$ cup (60 mL)	8
Sun-dried tomato, 1 cup (250 mL)	8
Milk, $1\frac{1}{4}$ cups (300 mL)	10
Eggs, 1 medium	6
Brown rice, cooked, 1 cup (250 mL)	5
Broccoli, cooked, 1 cup (250 mL)	4

Animal Sources of Protein

Meat Source	Grams of Protein Per Serving
Ground beef or steak, 3 oz (90 g)	27
Pork chop, 3 oz (90 g)	25
Turkey breast, 3 oz (90 g)	26
Tuna, 3 oz (90 g)	22
Chicken breast, 3 oz (90 g)	19
Salmon, cooked, 3 oz (90 g)	17

Associated Risk Factors

Diabetes Mellitus

Disorders of glucose (blood sugar) processing are strong predisposing factors toward fatty liver disease. These glucose disorders include type 2 diabetes mellitus (T2DM) and glucose intolerance. Type 2 diabetes is a disease characterized by excess sugars in the bloodstream. Insulin is a hormone synthesized by the pancreas and is responsible for maintaining proper blood sugar control. Insulin production and circulating amounts are generally preserved in T2DM. Insulin, however, does not function properly in this setting; it becomes resistant to its usual duties of managing sugars properly. Consequently, an elevated blood sugar is the end result.

FAQ

Q. **What is the difference between type 2 and type 1 diabetes?**

A. In type 1 diabetes, insulin deficiency is caused by an autoimmune phenomenon; in type 2 diabetes, insulin resistance typically arises from being overweight or obese.

Also known as juvenile diabetes, type 1 diabetes usually affects children and young adults. It arises due to an intrinsic problem of the pancreas — by not producing adequate amounts of insulin, resulting in insulin deficiency. In autoimmune diseases, your own immune system attacks various organs. People with autoimmune disease often have antibodies circulating in their system that perceive their own organs to be foreign objects. These antibodies attack various organs in an attempt to protect the body from a "foreign intruder." This is the case in type 1 diabetes. The patient produces antibodies that attack the pancreas, limiting production of insulin. Patients with type 1 diabetes are dependent on receiving insulin orally or intravenously from the time of diagnosis.

Insulin Resistance

Although type 1 diabetes is a risk factor for developing fatty liver disease, type 2 diabetes is the more serious contributing factor, mediated through insulin resistance. In this state of insulin resistance, insulin is present in appropriate amounts in the body but it does not work properly. Overweight and obesity is tightly linked to insulin resistance. Weight loss will lead to vastly improved sugar control and improved insulin function, ultimately resulting in the reduction of risk of developing heart disease and NAFLD.

High Triglycerides and Cholesterol

High triglyceride and cholesterol levels are well-established risk factors for the development of fatty liver disease. Patients must be in a fasting state when checking triglyceride and cholesterol levels.

Triglycerides

Triglycerides are the major form of fat stored by the body. A triglyceride molecule consists of three smaller fat molecules, called fatty acids, combined with a backbone made of alcohol glycerol. Our body produces some triglycerides, and others come from the food we eat. Triglyceride levels are influenced by recent fat and carbohydrate intake, as well as alcohol consumed. Elevated triglycerides are not only a risk factor for NAFLD, but also for heart disease.

Cholesterol

Cholesterol is a common type of steroid in the body. Cholesterol has developed a poor reputation because it is frequently associated with heart disease. However, cholesterol is critical to the formation of numerous hormones and vitamins, such as vitamin D, estrogens, progesterone, and cortisol. Cholesterol is carried in the blood as lipoproteins, which are a combination of fat and protein molecules.

The Bad and the Good

Low-density lipoprotein (LDL) is known as the "bad" cholesterol because elevated levels of LDL are associated with an increased risk of heart disease. Conversely, high-density lipoprotein (HDL) is the "good" cholesterol because higher levels of HDL are believed to protect against heart disease. Both high levels of LDL and low levels of HDL are risk factors for the development of fatty liver disease.

High Blood Pressure

High blood pressure, otherwise known as hypertension, is a common condition in which the force of the blood against the artery walls is high enough that it may eventually cause heart disease and damage to other organ systems, such as the kidney and brain, resulting in kidney failure or stroke. You can have high blood pressure for many years without any symptoms. For this reason, it is sometimes called the silent killer. High blood pressure can only be detected through routine measurements

---

DID YOU KNOW?

Ethnicity as a Risk Factor

Ethnicity has been noted to be a factor influencing the development of fatty liver disease, particularly in the United States. A higher prevalence of NAFLD predominates among Hispanics (45%) compared with Caucasians (33%) and African-Americans (24%). Certain subgroups of NAFLD can progress to more advanced forms of liver disease with greater frequency and rapidity than other groups. In Hispanic populations, the disease progresses more rapidly, for unknown reasons.

of blood pressure. It is easily detectable and, for the most part, easily treated through lifestyle changes and medications.

The Low and the High

Blood pressure readings consist of two numbers, the systolic and diastolic pressures. They are usually written one above the other. The top reading, or systolic pressure, refers to the pressure when your heart beats, pumping blood. The bottom number, or diastolic pressure, is the pressure when your heart is at rest, or in between beats. High blood pressure is defined as consistent readings greater than 140 over 90. In order to confirm a diagnosis of high blood pressure, serial measurements must be taken, separated by time. (Many people suffer from "white coat" hypertension, which is defined as high blood pressure seen in a doctor's office but not in other settings. This phenomenon is believed to arise due to anxiety that people experience during a clinic visit.) Hypertension is a risk factor for the development of fatty liver disease and should be managed meticulously not only in patients with known NAFLD, but also in all people with diagnosed high blood pressure.

Risk Factors for NAFLD
- Overweight and obesity
- Type 2 diabetes
- Elevated cholesterol and triglycerides
- High blood pressure
- Ethnicity
- Rapid weight loss, usually through weight loss surgery
- Total parenteral nutrition (artificial nutrition)

Metabolic Syndrome

The metabolic syndrome is a cluster of the most dangerous risk factors for heart disease:

- Abdominal obesity
- Type 2 diabetes
- High triglycerides and cholesterol
- High blood pressure

Due to the obesity epidemic in the developed world, the prevalence of the metabolic syndrome is quite high. A quarter of the world's population has the metabolic syndrome, and people with the metabolic syndrome are more than twice as likely to die from a heart attack or stroke compared to those without the syndrome. The metabolic syndrome is a strong risk factor for the development of NAFLD.

Although there are myriad additional risk factors for fatty liver disease, the majority of the risks for NAFLD arise from the metabolic syndrome. Your doctor will typically evaluate you for any additional risks, but in the majority of cases, treatment for NAFLD will usually be targeted on these metabolic risks.

Causes of Chronic Liver Disease
- Alcohol
- Hepatitis B and C, and other viruses
- Autoimmune hepatitis
- Hemochromatosis
- Wilson's disease
- Alpha 1-antitrypsin deficiency
- Primary biliary cirrhosis
- Primary sclerosing cholangitis
- Drugs

Chronic Liver Diseases

Fatty liver disease typically develops into a chronic liver condition if left undetected and untreated. Chronic liver disease from the following causes may be associated with fatty liver disease. These diseases can co-exist with fatty liver and must be ruled out prior to making a diagnosis of fatty liver disease.

Viral Hepatitis

The term "hepatitis" generally refers to liver inflammation. There are many viruses that can affect the liver, resulting in liver inflammation. The most common viruses that typically do this are hepatitis A, B, and C.

Hepatitis A

Hepatitis A affects about 150,000 people annually in the United States. Hepatitis A is an acute illness that never becomes chronic. This means that a patient with hepatitis A may become quite sick with jaundice, fatigue, muscle aches and pains, and flu-like symptoms for a period of time, and then spontaneously recover from these symptoms, with full recovery of the liver. However, most cases of hepatitis A run a much milder course.

Hepatitis A is typically transmitted through the fecal-oral route. This means that the virus is spread through ingestion of food or water that is contaminated by human waste containing hepatitis A. Hepatitis A may also be spread by kissing, handling oral secretions, and poor hand-washing. The risk factors for hepatitis A are quite different from those for hepatitis B or C. There is a vaccine available to prevent contraction of hepatitis A.

Hepatitis B

There are 300,000 new cases of hepatitis B in the United States each year. Hepatitis B is transmitted through blood or sexual contact. Risk factors for hepatitis B include blood transfusion with hepatitis-B-containing blood, accidental needle sticks with needles contaminated with hepatitis B, sexual contact with affected individuals, tattooing with contaminated needles, sharing razors and toothbrushes tainted with contaminated blood, and transmission of the virus from mother to baby at the time of delivery. There is a vaccine available to prevent contraction of hepatitis B.

Hepatitis C

Hepatitis C virus is another infection that affects the liver. Most people affected with hepatitis C don't even know they have it because hepatitis C quite rarely presents with symptoms. Hepatitis C is a chronic disease, which means most people who are not treated for it have the disease for life. Over time, infection with hepatitis C virus leads to scarring of the liver and ultimately cirrhosis.

People with hepatitis C often learn of their condition in a similar fashion to people affected with NAFLD, in that liver blood tests are performed for some other reason and are found to be elevated. When the hepatitis C antibody is positive on the blood test, the diagnosis of hepatitis C is confirmed. The risk factors that predispose an individual to hepatitis C are similar to those that predispose toward hepatitis B. These risk factors include blood-to-blood contact, usually through intravenous drug use or tainted blood transfusion. There is also a risk through unprotected sexual contact.

If hepatitis C is diagnosed, treatment for the virus may be offered, providing that the affected person meets all of the eligibility criteria. Treatment of hepatitis C has variable results depending on the subtype of the virus. The hepatitis C virus is divided in subtypes, known as genotypes. Genotypes 2 and 3 generally respond well to treatment, whereas the treatment response of genotype 1 virus is less robust. Your doctor will give you more details about the treatment options and the specific monitoring practices surrounding treatment if necessary.

> People with hepatitis C often learn of their condition in a similar fashion to people affected with NAFLD, in that liver blood tests are performed for some other reason and are found to be elevated.

Autoimmune Hepatitis

Autoimmune hepatitis is not a virus. Rather, it is a disease of the liver that occurs when your own immune system attacks the liver cells. This is an abnormal immune response that results in inflammation of the liver. Like hepatitis B and C, autoimmune hepatitis may lead to cirrhosis of the liver if left untreated. Autoimmune hepatitis is quite rare, affecting women more frequently than men.

Symptoms

The symptoms associated with autoimmune hepatitis are nonspecific, meaning that they may be seen with other diseases and not just autoimmune hepatitis. Some of these symptoms include fatigue, abdominal discomfort, joint pains, itching, yellowing of the skin (or jaundice), nausea, and vomiting. The diagnosis of autoimmune hepatitis is primarily made through more specific blood tests and liver biopsy. Once the diagnosis of autoimmune hepatitis is made, a referral to a gastroenterologist or hepatologist will be made and treatment will be initiated.

Hereditary Hemochromatosis

Hemochromatosis is a hereditary condition that results in an overload of iron. It is a condition that may affect many organs, not just the liver. Excess iron is deposited in organs, and this excess is responsible for the development of symptoms and disease. The typical organs and systems affected in hemochromatosis are the liver, heart, pancreas, joints, and skin, although the liver is the organ most frequently affected. Symptoms may arise as a consequence of involvement of each of these organs:

- When the heart is affected, symptoms of shortness of breath and swelling of the ankles may arise
- Involvement of the pancreas results in diabetes
- Involvement of the joints may lead to arthritis
- Involvement of the skin may lead to a darkening of pigmentation
- Involvement of the liver results in abnormal liver blood tests, but left untreated, hemochromatosis may result in liver cirrhosis

Where there is uncertainty about the diagnosis, a liver biopsy can provide confirmation of the diagnosis and provide valuable information about disease severity. Treatment of hemochromatosis in an otherwise healthy individual consists of regularly scheduled bloodletting, otherwise known as phlebotomy sessions. Your specialist will discuss the treatment options with you in detail when necessary.

Wilson's Disease

Wilson's disease is another hereditary, or genetic, disorder. It is caused by copper accumulation in various organs. The brain and liver are the two organs most frequently affected by excess copper deposition. The presence of liver disease from Wilson's disease may present either acutely or chronically. An acute manifestation of Wilson's disease may present with acute liver failure. This is a life-threatening condition where the liver fails to perform its routine duties, leading to waste accumulation in the bloodstream. When this occurs, you are vulnerable to confusion, seizures, coma, and death. Acute liver failure as a consequence of Wilson's disease occurs in 5% of patients affected with Wilson's disease. Chronic Wilson's disease may manifest as chronic hepatitis, or a chronically inflamed liver, which may result in cirrhosis over time.

Patients with chronic Wilson's disease affecting the liver often do not have any major symptoms. Symptoms generally develop only when the liver disease is advanced and cirrhotic. About half of people with Wilson's disease have neurological or psychiatric symptoms as a result of copper accumulation in the brain. These symptoms include mild memory impairment, clumsiness, and symptoms similar to those in Parkinson's disease (hand tremors, rigid and slow movements, slurred speech, and lack of coordination).

Diagnosis

The diagnosis of Wilson's disease is usually suspected based on abnormal blood and urine tests. The major copper-carrying protein in the blood, known as ceruloplasmin, is low in Wilson's disease, and a urine sample collected during a 24-hour period will show a high level of copper. Once the blood and urine tests indicate a suspicion for Wilson's disease, a liver biopsy is often done to confirm the diagnosis. Your specialist will discuss treatment options with you if you are diagnosed with Wilson's disease.

> About half of people with Wilson's disease have neurological or psychiatric symptoms as a result of copper accumulation in the brain.

Alpha 1-Antitrypsin Deficiency

Alpha 1-antitrypsin deficiency is a disease caused by the reduced production of the enzyme inhibitor alpha 1-antitrypsin. The role of alpha 1-antitrypsin is to protect the body tissues from the attack of certain enzymes. When alpha 1-antitrypsin levels are low, tissues in the lungs and liver are vulnerable to damage. Alpha 1-antitrypsin deficiency is an inherited condition. In the lungs, alpha 1-antitrypsin deficiency produces emphysema, which is a chronic lung disease. In the liver, alpha 1-antitrypsin deficiency may result in abnormal liver blood tests, liver scarring, and cirrhosis. The diagnosis is relatively easy to make. Alpha 1-antitrypsin levels can be measured in the blood. If the levels are low, then the diagnosis is confirmed. A liver biopsy may also be helpful in confirming the diagnosis and in assessing the severity of disease.

Primary Biliary Cirrhosis

Primary biliary cirrhosis (PBC) is an autoimmune disease of the liver. The liver is full of small bile ducts, which are responsible for clearing bile from the liver. PBC is caused by a destruction of the bile ducts, resulting in the buildup of bile in the liver. Over time, this can lead to scarring, fibrosis, and cirrhosis of the liver.

> PBC is caused by a destruction of the bile ducts, resulting in the buildup of bile in the liver. Over time, this can lead to scarring, fibrosis, and cirrhosis of the liver.

Symptoms seen with PBC include profound fatigue and itchiness of the skin, which can be extremely debilitating and severe, leading to depression, jaundice, and cirrhosis. The diagnosis of PBC is made from characteristic blood work, such as abnormal liver blood tests usually occurring in a specific type of pattern, and through the presence of certain antibodies. These typical antibodies, which are present in most cases of PBC, are anti-mitochondrial antibody (AMA) and antinuclear antibody (ANA). A liver biopsy can confirm the diagnosis and allow for assessment of severity, but it is not always routinely recommended in PBC. PBC can be managed efficiently with medications. One of the medications that has great value in treating PBC is ursodeoxycholic acid. Your specialist will discuss this in more detail with you if necessary.

Primary Sclerosing Cholangitis

Similar to PBC, primary sclerosing cholangitis (PSC) is a chronic liver disease caused by damage to the bile ducts. In contrast to PBC, PSC typically affects the larger bile ducts in the liver. These are general statements, however, and sometimes the small ducts are affected in PSC — although this occurs less frequently. Symptoms seen with PSC include fatigue, jaundice, itching, inadequate absorption of nutrients (particularly vitamins A, D, E, and K), and liver cirrhosis. Patients with PSC are likely to have an underlying diagnosis of either Crohn's disease or ulcerative colitis. The presence of PSC increases the likelihood of developing colon cancer in a patient who also has ulcerative colitis. PSC also increases the risk of developing cancer of the bile ducts, called cholangiocarcinoma. In contrast to PBC, PSC tends to affect men more frequently than women. PSC may be suspected through a routine liver ultrasound. However, an MRI of the liver is an excellent noninvasive method of confirming the diagnosis. A liver biopsy may be warranted in PSC to assess the severity of disease. Liver transplantation is the only proven long-term treatment of PSC.

Drug-Induced Liver Disease

Drug-induced liver diseases are caused by physician-prescribed medications, over-the-counter medications, vitamins, naturopathic remedies, hormones, and recreational drugs. Drugs can injure the liver in several ways. Some drugs are directly toxic to the liver, and other drugs may be transformed by the liver into chemicals that then are toxic to the liver. In some cases, drugs in low doses may not cause harm to the liver but will lead to liver injury if taken in high doses. In other cases, a drug may cause liver damage whether taken in low or high doses.

Drugs may cause many types of liver abnormalities. They may simply result in mild blood test abnormalities. However, the spectrum of drug-induced liver disease may progress to inflammation (hepatitis), fat accumulation, decreased bile flow, scarring, cirrhosis, and liver failure. There are many drugs that cause liver disease. I cannot stress too highly the importance of discussing your prescribed medications with your doctor if you are known to have liver disease, to ensure that your medications are not causing your liver disease or making the disease worse.

Drugs Associated with Fatty Liver Disease

- Steroids
- Tamoxifen (used for treatment of breast cancer)
- Amiodarone (used for heart arrhythmias)
- Diltiazem (used for high blood pressure)

Case History (continued)

John

Reviewing John's medical history, it becomes evident — with his obesity and high cholesterol and triglyceride levels — he is at risk for NAFLD. The chest pains are also quite concerning in consideration of heart disease. Therefore, it becomes imperative that appropriate investigations are taken not only to evaluate his liver disease further, but also to ensure that a complete cardiac assessment is undertaken.

Part 2

Managing Nonalcoholic Fatty Liver Disease

CHAPTER 4
Medications

Case History

William Barnes

William is a 52-year-old man who has NAFLD. He has high cholesterol and is obese. He has been trying to lose weight for years — unsuccessfully. He recently had a liver biopsy. When he came to our clinic for the results, I told him he had NASH (inflammation plus fibrosis) and that his risk of progressing to cirrhosis was moderate to high. He was quite dejected and frustrated. William admitted that weight loss has been quite challenging for him, and he asked me whether there was a pill he could take to help him with his NASH ...

(continued on page 53)

FAQ

Q. **Are there any medications that I can use to treat my NAFLD?**

A. Yes and no. There is a compelling need for researchers and scientists to continue investigating treatment options using medications. Many clinical trials have been conducted to determine the potential for drug therapy in managing this disease. Liver biopsy is the only known accurate method of determining whether or not any medication is having a positive impact on the underlying disease.

Lifestyle modifications focusing on dietary changes and exercise are the most important therapies for fatty liver disease, but lifestyle changes are hard to institute and even harder to maintain. Therefore, even if you are using medications to treat your condition, you should continue to make lifestyle modifications to handle your liver disease.

Anti-Diabetic Medications

In some cases, medications developed for treating type 2 diabetes have proven to be effective for managing fatty liver symptoms, especially if you have type 2 diabetes as well as NAFLD.

Metformin

Insulin resistance, a condition whereby insulin does not function effectively, is one of the primary mechanisms accounting for the onset of fatty liver disease. Insulin is a hormone produced by the pancreas, and it controls glucose levels in the blood by reducing the amount of glucose made by the liver and by increasing the removal of glucose from the blood by the muscle and fat tissue. Insulin resistance can be seen in the pre-diabetic state and in patients with diabetes. Agents that improve insulin resistance should potentially help patients with fatty liver disease. This class of medication is otherwise known as insulin sensitizers.

Metformin is known to many patients who suffer from diabetes. Metformin works by increasing the sensitivity of the liver, muscles, and fat so that sugar levels in the blood are reduced. Metformin has been evaluated in several small research studies in patients with NAFLD. Metformin has been shown to improve liver blood tests. However, when liver biopsies were performed, the effect of metformin in reducing NASH was seen as less robust. Many of these studies were quite short in duration. This means that an accurate assessment regarding the true effect of this medication cannot be made.

Side Effects

Metformin does have side effects that can be cumbersome to the patient. These side effects include nausea, vomiting, gas, bloating, and diarrhea. These symptoms can sometimes be severe enough to result in discontinuation of this treatment. There are also more serious side effects, including unusual muscle pain, weakness, trouble breathing, and an abnormal heartbeat. These more serious side effects are quite rare.

Pioglitazone

Pioglitazone falls in the thiazolidinedione (TZD) class of medications. TZDs also improve insulin resistance by allowing better utilization of insulin and glucose. The TZD class of medications has held promise in the treatment of NAFLD due to its beneficial impact on insulin resistance and metabolism of fatty acids in the liver. There are other medications in this class as well.

Side Effects

There are two drawbacks in using TZD medications. The first is the almost universal reversion of improvement after discontinuation of the drug, making it likely that long-term therapy with this medication is necessary. The second drawback is that pioglitazone use is associated with the side effects of leg swelling and weight gain of between 4 and 11 pounds (2 and 5 kg). This weight gain may limit the beneficial effects of this drug. The results from trials using TZDs for fatty liver disease do suggest some benefit, but the safety of this medication, in part mediated by the side effects, is currently unknown. At this time, TZDs should only be reserved for second-line treatment and possibly for patients with diabetes and NAFLD. Ask your doctor for further information about this medication.

At this time, TZDs should only be reserved for second-line treatment and possibly for patients with diabetes and NAFLD.

Lipid-Lowering Medications

There are a number of medications currently used to manage high triglycerides and cholesterol, which are collectively known as lipids. Perhaps the best-known of these lipid-lowering drugs are the statins, a class of drugs that lower the levels of cholesterol in the blood by reducing the production of cholesterol in the liver. Statins block the enzyme in the liver that is responsible for making cholesterol.

High lipid levels are a major risk factor for fatty liver disease. Addressing high cholesterol levels should theoretically induce improvement in NAFLD, and there have been some clinical trials evaluating the effects of this class of medications in patients with NAFLD. None of the studies, however, showed improvement in the fibrosis (scarring) component of NAFLD. However, one study did show that patients receiving statins had less fat accumulation in their liver and had a slower rate of progression toward scarring of the liver.

High lipid levels are a major risk factor for fatty liver disease. Addressing high cholesterol levels should theoretically induce improvement in NAFLD, and there have been some clinical trials evaluating the effects of this class of medications in patients with NAFLD.

Intrinsic Liver Injury

One of the major concerns with this class of medications is that of intrinsic liver injury from the medication itself. A medication in this class can cause liver failure, independent of any other liver disease. This fear has caused great concern among physicians, and many have been reticent to prescribe statins to people with underlying liver problems. However, a number of large studies have now demonstrated the safety of statins in patients with underlying NAFLD and abnormal cholesterol and triglyceride levels. In these patients, statins are an important part of the management of their risk factors for heart disease and fatty liver disease.

Antioxidant Agents

Oxidative stress is believed to play a role in the development of fatty liver disease. Oxidative stress is caused by an imbalance between the production of highly reactive oxygen and the ability of the liver to readily detoxify these oxygen particles. Disturbances or imbalances in this system lead to damaged cells, proteins, and even DNA particles, and they predispose you toward several diseases, such as heart disease, Parkinson's disease, cancer, and fatty liver disease.

Examples of Lipid-Lowering Statin Medications
- Atorvastatin (Lipitor)
- Fluvastatin (Lescol)
- Lovastatin (Mevacor)
- Pravastatin (Pravachol)
- Rosuvastatin (Crestor)
- Simvastatin (Zocor)

Vitamin E

There have been medical studies evaluating the effects of a few types of antioxidant medications in NAFLD. The best of these studies has involved vitamin E. Vitamin E is a fat-soluble vitamin and a potent antioxidant. Vitamin E treatment has been shown to result in improvement in the liver biopsy findings in NAFLD. These results are quite promising and suggest that patients with NAFLD may benefit from consistent use. However, this information must be balanced by the concerns regarding the long-term safety of vitamin E. In some studies, doses in excess of 400 IUs daily have been associated with an increase in death from all causes, although this has been inconsistently reported.

FAQ

Q. Should I be taking vitamin E supplements to manage my fatty liver disease?

A. Before taking vitamin E therapeutically, it is generally recommended that patients first have a liver biopsy to assess the severity of their disease and that they make lifestyle modifications that result in improvement of liver blood tests. If the liver biopsy results show convincing evidence of NASH (fat plus inflammation), vitamin E at a dose of 800 IUs daily can be helpful in some patients. However, do not self-prescribe vitamin E. Talk to your doctor about this approach prior to supplementation.

Silymarin

Silymarin, otherwise known as milk thistle, is an extract from the *Silybum marianum* plant. Its use among patients with liver disease is popular because it is viewed as a "natural" substance and to date has not been associated with significant adverse side effects. There has been one very small study that suggested some improvement in liver blood tests; however, well-designed medical studies showing benefit from this agent are lacking. Additionally, there is a lack of standardization of silymarin in the available formulations. For these reasons, silymarin is generally not recommended for patients with NAFLD.

Anti-Obesity Drugs

Drug treatments for obesity would appear to be a promising option for patients with fatty liver disease. However, drug therapy for obesity has not shown a direct beneficial effect on the liver independent of weight loss. This means that drug therapy for obesity that results in modest weight loss has a beneficial impact on the liver, but drug therapy for weight loss that does not have the desired effect on weight does not help the liver.

Case History (continued)

William

I reiterated to William that there is no quick fix for NAFLD, and that he must continue with dietary modifications and the incorporation of regular physical activity into his week. However, because he also has abnormal cholesterol, he would benefit from a lipid-lowering agent, and I suggested a statin for him. I told William that there was a modest likelihood the statin would have a positive impact on his liver. However, I did mention that statin use was associated with rare cases of liver failure, and I suggested that he monitor his liver enzymes more regularly in the initial phases of using this drug. Because his liver biopsy confirmed that William has NASH, we had a discussion surrounding the risks and benefits of using vitamin E. William did not have a strong family history of heart disease, and he was not a smoker. Therefore, we made the decision to start vitamin E as part of his therapy. William was aware of the controversies surrounding possible increased mortality due to vitamin E; however, this was balanced by the risk of developing liver cirrhosis.

CHAPTER 5

Physical Activity and Exercise

Case History

Carolyn Lynch

Carolyn is a 38-year-old woman who was diagnosed with NAFLD 5 years ago. She has weighed 250 pounds (113 kg) consistently for the past 5 years, with a BMI of 35 (class 2 obesity), despite numerous attempts at dieting. In fact, she had followed both the Bernstein diet program and Weight Watchers program at different points during the past 5 years, but she was unsuccessful at losing weight. She has been quite frustrated at her dieting experience and wonders what more she could do to help her NAFLD. To help with her frustration, Carolyn had started deep-water running and aqua fitness. She has been doing this now for the past year. Although she has not lost any weight, her gastroenterologist told her during her most recent visit that her liver blood tests had improved considerably and are now back to normal. Carolyn was delighted at this news but wonders how her NAFLD could be so much better when she hadn't lost any weight ...

(continued on page 58)

For years, weight loss has been the mainstay of therapy for the treatment of fatty liver disease, and weight loss has been seen as the result of dietary modifications and an increase in activities and exercise that burn excess calories stored as fat in the body. Although physical activity and exercise do not necessarily lead to weight loss, regular exercise can improve the course of NAFLD substantially. "Physical activity" and "exercise," although used interchangeably, do not refer to the same thing.

Physical Activity

"Physical activity" refers to activity that is part of your daily life. Household, workplace, and lifestyle physical activity are three of the most common types of physical activity. Examples of household physical activity include sweeping and cleaning; workplace activities include lifting boxes and delivering packages as a bike courier; and lifestyle physical activities include carrying a basket at the grocery store (rather than wheeling a cart) or doing the housework yourself.

Exercise

Exercise is a form of physical activity that is planned or structured to improve at least one aspect of physical fitness — endurance, strength, or flexibility. Regular physical fitness exercise can have a positive impact on fatty liver disease.

Kinds of Exercise
- Endurance (aerobic)
- Strength (resistance)
- Flexibility (stretching)

Benefits

Visceral Adipose Tissue (VAT) Reduction

Regular exercise may result in an improvement in NAFLD independent of weight loss. The fat located in the abdomen is divided into two separate compartments: the visceral adipose tissue, otherwise known as VAT, and subcutaneous adipose tissue, known as SAT. VAT is the fat tissue located immediately surrounding the internal organs. SAT is the fat tissue located immediately beneath the skin.

VAT

VAT secretes hormones that have toxic properties into the body, leading to increased inflammation and disease severity. Exercise has been shown to reduce the VAT component of fat. In fact, exercise reduces the VAT fat component to a much greater degree than weight loss achieved through diet could ever hope to.

Increased Muscle Mass

Another benefit of regular exercise is an increase in muscle mass. Muscle burns calories. The presence of more muscle generally translates into a greater number of calories burned. One of the major goals of exercise is to build muscle weight that will help in burning calories, contributing toward weight loss. Both endurance (aerobic) and strength (resistance) exercise have been shown to have favorable effects in patients with fatty liver disease.

Favorable Impact on Glucose

Glucose intolerance and diabetes predispose you to NAFLD. Exercise has been shown to improve blood glucose levels, and many cases of type 2 diabetes have resolved through exercise alone. Exercise is an essential part of the treatment of diabetes. It can reduce the need for any diabetes medication, and it can reduce the need for insulin therapy in many patients with type 2 diabetes. Patients who have had diabetes for many years are at risk for complications from diabetes. These complications include chronic kidney disease that may result in kidney failure (requiring dialysis), heart attack, stroke, and blindness, just to mention a few. Regular exercise can maintain blood sugars in the appropriate ranges, limiting these unwanted complications.

Lipid-Lowering Effects

High triglyceride and cholesterol levels are risk factors for heart disease and heart attacks. High triglyceride and cholesterol levels also predispose you toward NAFLD, and — if untreated — can have an unfavorable impact on NAFLD. Regular exercise can maintain triglyceride and cholesterol values in good ranges, reducing the impact on fatty liver disease.

Additional Benefits of Exercise

Exercise can reduce the risk of many other health problems. Additional benefits of exercise include a reduction in the risk of:

- Dying prematurely
- Developing heart disease
- Developing high blood pressure
- Developing colon cancer

Exercise also reduces feelings of anxiety and depression, improves blood pressure control in people previously diagnosed with high blood pressure, and helps build and maintain healthy bones, muscles, and joints. Regular exercise promotes decreased fat content in the liver, improves the risk of heart disease, and protects against diabetes regardless of weight loss.

Exercise Goals

Regular moderate exercise should be implemented by all patients with NAFLD who are capable of engaging in a structured exercise program. People lead busy lives, and it's easy to see why scheduling regular physical activity or exercise is challenging. However, every time you think about exercise but feel too tired or overcommitted in other aspects of your life, think about the numerous health benefits afforded by exercise — and get moving!

Endurance (Aerobic) Goals

In accordance with the Canadian physical activity guidelines published by the Canadian Society for Exercise Physiology, adults 18 to 64 years of age should accumulate at least 150 minutes of moderate- to vigorous-intensity aerobic physical activity weekly, in bouts of at least 10 minutes or more.

Strength (Resistance) Goals

It is also beneficial to add muscle mass by working the major muscle groups. Moderate-intensity physical activities will result in mild to moderate perspiration and a faster rate of breathing. Vigorous-intensity physical activities will result in dripping perspiration and a sensation of being completely out of breath.

Activity and Exercise Program

Here are some basic tips to encourage a regular exercise and activity routine.

1. Choose a variety of physical activities you enjoy. Try different activities until you find the ones right for you.
2. Get into a routine. Try to go to the pool or gym, or join a group exercise class, at the same time each day. Plan ahead. Consider bringing a friend, which will increase accountability and help ensure your follow-through with the designated activity.
3. Limit the time you spend watching television or sitting in front of a computer during your leisure time.
4. Take the "harder" modality of transportation when possible. Walk, bike, or jog instead of driving.
5. Join a team activity. You'll make new friends and be active at the same time.
6. Set a goal, make a plan, pick a time and place, and remember that every step counts!

> **DID YOU KNOW?**
>
> **Compounded Effect**
>
> Both resistance exercise and aerobic exercise can result in an improvement in NAFLD; however, combined resistance and aerobic exercise appears to be superior in achieving a greater impact in NAFLD than either modality alone.

Carolyn

After obtaining further history from Carolyn, it became evident that she was determined to change her lifestyle and engage in regular routine exercise, although she still struggled with many responsibilities demanding her attention. She had joined aqua fit for twice weekly, but she only ended up going once a week because the class coincided with the time her children needed to be picked up from school. Carolyn did some research and found out that there was an evening class just after supper. Carolyn's husband chipped in to do evening duty with the family one night a week, and that gesture allowed Carolyn to get to her second class of aqua fit, which she really enjoyed doing. She believed in dedicating this time toward improving her health and self-worth. In fact, she encouraged her teenage daughter to join her, enhancing quality time with her daughter.

CHAPTER 6

Weight Loss Therapy

Case History

Karla Castenade

Karla is a 32-year-old woman who was an overweight teenager and is now an obese adult. She weighs 190 pounds (86 kg) and is five foot three (160 cm). She has been frustrated about her weight for most of her adult life and has tried almost every "fad" diet to counteract her diabetes and NAFLD. Moreover, Karla has a strong family history of heart disease and was determined to do what was necessary to reduce her risk of developing the same. About 10 years ago, she followed the Atkins diet for a total of 12 weeks. In the first few weeks, Karla lost 10 pounds (5 kg)! She was ecstatic with that result. However, during the fourth week of the diet, Karla started having headaches and an unexplained loss of energy. She felt quite lethargic. By week six, Karla was struggling, trying to find food choices that fit with her personality and her unique preferences. She loved bread and pastas, and craved certain vegetables that were largely forbidden from this diet. She started to make food choices that were not in line with this dietary plan. At the 8-week mark, Karla started to regain the weight she had previously lost. By week 12, she had returned back to her original weight.

Karla has also tried the South Beach diet. Karla did experience modest weight loss; however, she found that she often craved certain foods that were high on the glycemic index (described below). When she would indulge in these foods, Karla felt quite guilty and didn't know how to get back on track. Moreover, she wanted to exercise, but she didn't know how to get started or how to monitor her activity. Karla is currently following the Weight Watchers program. She feels that the holistic approach is exactly what she needs ...

(continued on page 75)

The main treatment goals of fatty liver disease mirror those of obesity. Addressing the primary issue of obesity will result in desirable consequences for the liver. Obesity is a very heterogeneous condition, so please keep in mind that there is no single strategy that will result in consistent benefits for all people. At present, there is no uniform cure for obesity. Any successful plan will involve a commitment to long-term, consistent lifestyle modifications, with an enabling support group of family and friends and an intrinsic desire to succeed.

Weight Loss Maintenance Challenge

The majority of people with obesity who have gone through the process of weight loss will tell you that losing weight is not the real battle. The real battle lies in the maintenance of weight loss. The primary reason for this is that there is no substitute for a commitment to lifestyle changes. Unless you can commit to the long haul of maintaining a certain lifestyle, success will be limited. It is necessary to be comfortable and confident with the lifestyle that you adopt to lose weight. When this has been accepted and implemented, you will likely be able to persist with that lifestyle to maintain weight loss.

Weight Loss Treatment Goals

Treatment goals must be realistic and focus on improving health status and quality of life — rather than focusing on the number on the scale. Specifically, with regard to fatty liver disease, the main goal is to lose 5% to 10% of baseline weight. Realistically, for most individuals, 5% to 10% of weight loss is feasible with some lifestyle modifications. In many cases, altering body composition to favor lean muscle over fat mass is sufficient to improve the consequences on the liver. This is generally achieved through regular structured exercise. If this is achieved, you may not see a change in the numbers on the scale, but your liver tests will improve, as will other critical parameters, such as blood sugar and blood pressure.

Moderate Weight Loss

Sometimes people overestimate the amount of weight loss necessary to be successful. Very modest amounts of weight loss can have health benefits. For example, if you are a 225-pound (102 kg) woman and have a BMI of 35 (class 2 obesity), your weight loss goals to induce an improvement on your liver — as well as on your heart health, diabetes, and blood pressure — lie between 10 and 25 pounds (5 and 11 kg)! In this situation, your goal is not to get back to your high school weight of 120 pounds (54 kg), although this might be your preconception. With this bit of information in mind, doesn't is suddenly seem more feasible and attainable to lose 20 pounds (10 kg) instead of 100 pounds (50 kg)?

DID YOU KNOW?

Weight Cycling

One of the main barriers to consistent success with weight loss is a constant battle with weight cycling. Weight cycling is characterized by periods of successful weight loss followed by remission and relapse that results in weight gain. The impact of weight cycling on health remains controversial; however, there is some medical evidence that suggests weight cycling results in increased body fat, which impairs subsequent weight loss efforts.

Restricting and Burning Calories

Weight loss is achieved by expending more energy than you consume, either by eating less or exercising more — or both. If you eat more calories than you consume, you will likely gain weight. An excess of 3500 calories consumed over calories expended results in a weight gain of 1 pound (500 g) of fat. To lose that weight, you will need to expend an extra 3500 calories. This can be done gradually. Consuming 500 fewer calories daily for 1 week will result in a 1-pound (500 g) weight loss at the end of that week.

Generally speaking, successful weight loss programs promote weight loss at a rate of 1 to 2 pounds (500 g to 1 kg) weekly. Diets that promote and guarantee more rapid results in weight loss are generally much more restrictive and are less likely to promote long-term adherence and facilitate success. In most cases, a combination of lifestyle changes — including eating behaviors, foods consumed, regular physical activity, medications, and/or surgery — will increase the likelihood of weight maintenance.

FAQ

Q. **What is a calorie?**

A. A calorie is a unit of heat energy. Heat energy is what fuels our body, just like gasoline fuels a car. All foods consist of calories waiting to be activated when you digest them. Calories are provided by three macronutrients: fat, carbohydrate, and protein. Fats have 9 calories per gram of pure fat, and protein and carbohydrates each have 4 calories per gram of pure protein or pure carbohydrate. The average male needs 2200 calories daily to remain healthy, and the average female needs 2000 calories. Physical activities and exercise burn these calories. You can use a calorie calculator to calculate how many calories you eat in a meal. They are based on the kind of food you consume and the serving size. Ask your dietitian for help in calculating you daily calorie intake — and expenditure.

Popular Diets

A number of popular diets claim to promote weight loss and weight maintenance. Popular "fad" diets generally promote short-term weight loss, usually with no concern for long-term weight maintenance. Losing a lot of weight in a short period of time is actually quite detrimental to the liver and can make the underlying fatty liver problem worse! Additionally, weight loss in the short term without any strategy in place for long-term weight maintenance is not helpful for your long-term health. There are a number of fad diets that have been popularized over the years. From a health perspective, exercise caution if you embark on a fad diet for the purpose of weight loss or to help any underlying health concern.

How To Spot a Fad Diet
A fad diet:

1. Makes claims that sound too good to be true.
2. Promises fast weight loss.
3. Does not encourage long-term diet and exercise lifestyle changes or provide a weight maintenance plan.
4. Recommends consuming less than 1000 calories daily.
5. Eliminates a complete food group (grains, fats, meats, vegetables, dairy).
6. Suggests you purchase only their products and does not teach you how to make healthy choices from a grocery store.
7. Lacks scientific medical studies proving that the diet works in a safe manner. Although many diets may claim that research studies show efficacy and safety, many of these studies were not conducted using an adequate number of people and were not subject to good and rigorous study methods.

Please talk to your dietitian if you plan to try any of these diet plans for the purpose of weight loss.

Three of the most popular weight loss diets are the Atkins diet, the South Beach diet, and the Weight Watchers program.

Atkins Diet
The Atkins diet is one of the best-known fad diets. It is a high-protein, high-fat, and low-carbohydrate plan. This diet has been around for many years and has undergone many revisions. In its most current format, the Atkins diet consists of four phases.

Four Phases
Phase One
Phase one, also known as the induction phase, severely restricts carbohydrates, limiting your intake to only 20 grams of

Fad Diets
- Atkins diet
- Cabbage soup diet
- Grapefruit diet
- Slim-Fast diet
- South Beach diet
- Zone diet

Atkins Diet
- High protein consumption
- High fat consumption
- Low carbohydrate consumption

carbohydrates daily. However, there is no suggested restriction on the consumption of fats or proteins. One concern with this diet plan is that followers can eat quite large amounts of fats during not only this induction phase, but during all phases of this diet, which can carry some serious health consequences. Generally, the induction phase lasts 2 weeks.

Phase Two

This phase introduces new foods and restores more types of food, including carbohydrates. However, the recommended carbohydrate intake during phase two is still quite low, around 40 grams daily. People who follow this diet are encouraged to continue this limited carbohydrate intake until they are within 10 pounds (5 kg) of their goal weight. Once they meet this criterion, they can advance to phase three of the program.

Phase Three

During this phase, people who follow this diet can gradually add 10 grams of carbohydrates weekly. Weight loss in this phase will slow down and soon plateau.

Phase Four

This is a weight maintenance phase, whereby followers achieve a certain carbohydrate level that sustains weight maintenance.

Evaluation

The Atkins diet can deliver effective weight loss, but the cost of restricting carbohydrates can have long-term health consequences with an impact on the course of fatty liver disease.

Fat Focus

There is no doubt that following a severely carbohydrate-restricted diet will result in weight loss in the short term. This is primarily due to allowing your body an opportunity to shift from burning carbohydrates for energy to burning stored fat. Typically, your body will burn the carbohydrates you eat for fuel until the carbohydrate sources are exhausted, and then it will burn fat. However, if there are minimal carbohydrates available from your diet, your body will burn fat sooner, resulting in fat loss.

DID YOU KNOW?

Water Loss

It is important to note that the Atkins diet claims that followers experience a relatively substantial weight loss in the initial stages of the diet. This is true. However, a lot of this weight loss will come from water weight, rather than fat weight. Most diets that claim rapid weight loss in a short period of time usually achieve this by encouraging water loss, or a diuretic effect. Rapid weight loss is defined as weight loss greater than 2 pounds (1 kg) weekly. Rapid water loss is not desirable and may affect the electrolytes, or salts, in your body, in addition to leaving you devoid of energy and feeling lethargic.

Carbohydrate Starvation

Adhering to the prescribed 20 grams and 40 grams of carbohydrates daily can be challenging at best. Human brains require at least 100 grams of carbohydrate daily for normal function. Restriction of carbohydrates to less than this value may lead to memory problems and slower cognition.

Micronutrient Deficiency

Additionally, many of the restricted foods are quite rich in the nutrients that are protective to the body on a number of different levels. These foods are rich in fiber and antioxidants, and they provide a number of other micronutrients not readily available through other food groups. By limiting these foods, followers risk missing out on critical nutrients responsible for health and wellness. Although it is probably quite feasible to limit carbohydrate intake to these levels in the short term, long-term adherence to this strategy is seldom successful.

Carbohydrate Quantity of Common Foods

Whole Grains	Serving	Carbohydrates (grams)
Bread, whole wheat	1 slice	14
Bread, multigrain	1 slice	17
Bread, rye	1 slice	15
Oatmeal, cooked	1 cup (250 mL)	25
Pancake, buckwheat mix	$\frac{1}{3}$ cup (75 mL) (3 cakes)	33
Pancake, whole-grain mix	$\frac{1}{3}$ cup (75 mL) (3 cakes)	28
Pasta, whole wheat, cooked	1 cup (250 mL)	37
Popcorn, popped	$3\frac{1}{2}$ cups (875 mL)	19
Rice, basmati brown, dry	$\frac{1}{4}$ cup (60 mL)	31
Rice, brown, cooked	$\frac{1}{2}$ cup (125 mL)	22
Rice, brown, dry	$\frac{1}{4}$ cup (60 mL)	33
Rice, wild, cooked	$\frac{1}{2}$ cup (125 mL)	18

Fruits (raw)	Amount	Carbohydrates (grams)
Apple	5 oz (150 g)	21
Avocado	½ (3 oz/90 g)	7
Blackberries	1 cup (250 mL)	18
Blueberries	1 cup (250 mL)	21
Cantaloupe	1 cup (250 mL)	13
Cranberries	½ cup (125 mL)	6
Grapefruit	½ (4 oz/125 g)	10
Grapes	1 cup (250 mL)	16
Guava	1 (3 oz/90 g)	11
Kiwi	1 (2½ oz/75 g)	11
Mango	½ (3½ oz/105 g)	18
Nectarine	1 (5 oz/150 g)	16
Orange	1 (4½ oz/140 g)	15
Papaya	½ (5½ oz/165 g)	15
Peach	1 (3½ oz/105 g)	10
Pear	1 (6 oz/175 g)	25
Pineapple	1 cup (250 mL)	19
Raspberries	1 cup (250 mL)	14
Strawberries	1 cup (250 mL)	11
Tangerine	1 (3 oz/90 g)	9
Watermelon	1 cup (250 mL)	12

Beans and Peas	Amount	Carbohydrates (grams)
Black beans, cooked	½ cup (125 mL)	18
Black beans, dry	¼ cup (60 mL)	23
Chickpeas, cooked	½ cup (125 mL)	18
Chickpeas, dry	¼ cup (60 mL)	28
Kidney beans, cooked	½ cup (125 mL)	20

Beans and Peas	Amount	Carbohydrates (grams)
Kidney beans, dry	¼ cup (60 mL)	29
Lentils, cooked	½ cup (125 mL)	20
Lentils, dry	¼ cup (60 mL)	28
Lima beans, cooked	½ cup (125 mL)	20
Lima beans, dry	¼ cup (60 mL)	22
Navy beans, cooked	½ cup (125 mL)	29
Navy beans, dry	¼ cup (60 mL)	32
Pinto beans, cooked	½ cup (125 mL)	22
Pinto beans, dry	¼ cup (60 mL)	29
Soybeans, cooked	½ cup (125 mL)	9
Soybeans, dry	¼ cup (60 mL)	13
Split peas, cooked	½ cup (125 mL)	21
Split peas, dry	¼ cup (60 mL)	26

Vegetables	Amount	Carbohydrates (grams)
Alfalfa sprouts, raw	½ cup (125 mL)	1
Asparagus, cooked	½ cup (125 mL)	4
Bell peppers, green, raw	½ cup (125 mL)	3
Bell peppers, red, raw	½ cup (125 mL)	3
Broccoli, cooked	½ cup (125 mL)	4
Brussels sprouts, cooked	½ cup (125 mL)	7
Cabbage, cooked	½ cup (125 mL)	4
Carrot, cooked	1 (2½ oz/75 g)	7
Cauliflower, cooked	3 florets	3
Celery, raw	½ cup (125 mL)	2
Cabbage, Chinese, cooked	½ cup (125 mL)	2
Cabbage, red, cooked	½ cup (125 mL)	4
Chile peppers	1 tbsp (15 mL)	1

Vegetables	Amount	Carbohydrates (grams)
Corn (sweet)	1 ear	19
Cucumber, raw	5 oz (150 g)	4
Edamame (fresh soybeans), raw	½ cup (125 mL)	14
Edamame, cooked	¼ cup (60 mL)	10
Eggplant, cooked	½ cup (125 mL)	3
Garlic	1 clove	1
Gingerroot, raw	1 tbsp (15 mL)	1
Lettuce, butterhead, raw	1 cup (250 mL)	2
Lettuce, iceberg, raw	1½ cups (375 mL)	3
Lettuce, romaine, raw	1½ cups (375 mL)	2
Mushrooms, cooked	½ cup (125 mL)	4
Okra, cooked	½ cup (125 mL)	6
Onions, cooked	½ cup (125 mL)	7
Radishes, raw	½ cup (125 mL)	2
Scallions, raw	½ cup (125 mL)	4
Spinach, cooked	½ cup (125 mL)	3
Swiss chard, cooked	½ cup (125 mL)	4
Zucchini, cooked	½ cup (125 mL)	4

South Beach Diet

The South Beach diet advocates replacing "bad carbohydrates" with "good carbohydrates" and replacing "bad fats" with "good fats." Similar to the Atkins diet, the South Beach diet has several phases, the first promising rapid weight loss, which is likely due to water loss (not fat loss). Specific carbohydrates are restricted in the first phase of the diet, with an increase in variety in the next phases.

"Bad" Carbohydrates and Fats

Carbohydrate-rich foods, which the body digests quickly, usually result in a spike in blood sugar. Foods that can cause these blood sugar spikes generally contain refined sugars and grains, which comprise a large part of the Western diet. The South Beach diet recommends eliminating these refined carbohydrates in favor of relatively unprocessed foods, such as vegetables, beans, and whole grains.

According to the South Beach diet, carbohydrates are considered "good" only if they have a low glycemic index. The repetitive consumption of foods higher on the glycemic index can lead to rapid bursts of insulin secreted from the pancreas, with the risk of "burning out" the pancreas, resulting in diabetes. Medical studies have shown that people who follow a low glycemic index diet for a substantive period of time are at lower risk for developing diabetes, heart disease, and obesity.

FAQ

Q. **What is the glycemic index?**

A. The glycemic index (GI) is a measure of the effects that carbohydrates have on blood sugar levels. It estimates how much each gram of available carbohydrate in a food raises a person's blood glucose level following ingestion of the food, relative to the consumption of glucose. By definition, glucose has a glycemic index of 100. Foods with carbohydrates that break down quickly during digestion and release glucose rapidly into the bloodstream (like simple sugars and refined products) have a higher glycemic index. Foods with carbohydrates that break down more slowly, releasing glucose more gradually into the bloodstream, have a lower glycemic index and result in more optimally controlled blood sugars. These foods — minimally processed grains, whole fruits, legumes, nuts, and vegetables — are much better for patients with diabetes.

Glycemic Index Ranges

- Lower glycemic index foods have a glycemic index range of less than 55.
- Medium glycemic index foods have a glycemic index range between 56 and 69.
- High glycemic index foods have a glycemic index range higher than 70.

The South Beach diet also recommends avoidance of "bad" fats. These bad fats include trans fats and saturated fats. Replacing these bad fats with foods rich in unsaturated fats and omega-3 fats is recommended.

Evaluation

The South Beach diet was initially developed by cardiologist Arthur Agatston to assist patients with weight loss in order to lower their risk of developing heart disease, to obtain better control of their diabetes, and to provide ownership of their health. Some have criticized this diet with regard to inconsistent benefits on all of these fronts.

Nevertheless, there are many positive attributes to the South Beach diet, especially in showing how to choose good carbohydrates and good fats. However, it is important to be cautious of rapid weight loss in the early phases of this diet because this may worsen your fatty liver condition and may leave you feeling weak and tired due to dehydration. Prior to embarking on this diet, consult with your health-care provider to discuss the positive and negative health attributes of this diet plan.

Glycemic Index of Common Foods

Classification	GI range	Examples	
Low GI	55 or lower	• Most fruits and vegetables (excluding those below) • Legumes and pulses • Some whole, intact grains • Beets	• Chickpeas • Kidney beans • Nuts • Fructose • Tagatose
Medium GI	56–69	• Basmati rice • Cranberry juice • Grapes • Ice cream • Pita bread	• Pumpernickel bread • Raisins • Whole wheat products • Sucrose
High GI	70 and higher	• Corn flakes • Extruded breakfast cereals • Most white rices • Pretzels • White bread	• White potato • Glucose • Maltodextrin • Maltose

Weight Watchers

The Weight Watchers weight loss program is arguably the best-known program for weight loss. It was first launched in the early 1960s. The Weight Watchers program is committed to providing a comprehensive approach to weight loss, and it is based on the evolution of the science of overweight conditions and obesity.

The Weight Watchers weight loss program is arguably the best-known program for weight loss. It was first launched in the early 1960s.

Weight Loss Principles

There are four principles that guide the philosophy of the Weight Watchers program, and they are based on good scientific evidence. This program is effective for most individuals and it is safe.

1. *Weight loss:* Participants can expect weight loss of up to 2 pounds (1 kg) per week.
2. *Diet:* The diet includes food choices that not only restrict calories but also meet scientific recommendations for nutritional completeness, with reduction in the risk of many disease states.
3. *Exercise:* The program advocates an activity plan that concurrently provides the complete range of weight- and health-related benefits that are associated with exercise.
4. *Commitment:* This is a program for committed individuals and one that is sustainable in the long term. Short-term weight loss for reduction in health risk is not the desired outcome for people with health-related disease. Weight loss that is maintained in the long term is the desirable outcome, and one that the Weight Watchers program is committed to providing.

Weight loss that is maintained in the long term is the desirable outcome, and one that the Weight Watchers program is committed to providing.

Food Choices

The Weight Watchers program endorses some fundamental food choices that are essential for good health and nutrition.

1. Eat at least 5 servings of fruits and vegetables daily.
2. Drink at least 2 servings of milk daily for adults between the ages of 18 and 50; nursing women, teenagers, and people over the age 50 should consume 3 servings daily.
3. Drink at least 6 glasses of water daily.
4. Consume at least 1 to 2 servings of protein-rich foods.
5. Limit added sugars, sodium, and alcohol.
6. Choose whole-grain foods whenever possible.

Evaluation

- *Practical*: The Weight Watchers program is realistic and practical. It can be incorporated into almost any person's busy lifestyle.
- *Flexible*: It is also relatively flexible, so that people can apply the approaches they learn through the program into their daily routines.
- *Informative*: Patients like to be informed regarding the "why" behind their doctor's recommendations. An educated patient is often the most successful in following a challenging diet and lifestyle program. Explaining not only what to do but also why empowers people, and it provides them with the tools they need to move forward in enriching their health. The Weight Watchers program educates individuals who follow this program, and provides them with an understanding and the confidence necessary to persist with lifestyle changes to ensure success.

PointsPlus Program

When it comes to food choices and preferences, we are all quite unique. A prescriptive approach, or a one-size-fits-all approach, is prone to failure, and it can breed a sense of frustration — especially if that approach is diametrically opposite to a food approach that brings you satisfaction as a unique individual. To prescribe a low-carbohydrate diet to a lover of pastas and bread, for example, is likely going to meet with failure. Weight loss success depends on finding a method that fits within one's lifestyle and preferences. The Weight Watchers program offers a PointsPlus program that has foundations in a simple-to-learn, flexible counting system. This system helps guide people toward healthier, more satisfying food choices without demanding strict adherence to any food restrictions.

Numerical values

The general idea of the PointsPlus program is that every food and drink has a numerical value. This number is derived from a formula that uses the nutritional characteristics of that particular food item; it takes into consideration the major nutrients of carbohydrate, fat, protein, and fiber; and it factors in how satisfying each of these nutrients is for the dieter. For example, foods rich in protein and fiber are more satisfying than fat and non-fiber-rich carbohydrates. These foods are generally lower in points. By allocating foods to a certain point value, the need to weigh and measure foods precisely is eliminated, and it instead encourages a focus on the bigger picture by building awareness of food choices — and the health benefits or adverse consequences that go along with those choices. The total of allowable points that may be consumed daily is based on your current weight, sex, height, and age.

Flexible restraint

This program also imparts the skill of flexible restraint. This is the ability to apply a moderate level of control on eating behaviors and patterns, which is important to weight loss success. The key is to find the balance between self-control and flexibility in an eating plan that is relatively easy to follow. To help with developing this skill, the PointsPlus program provides a system that allows for eating treats in a controlled manner, without sacrificing weight loss.

Behavioral change

Any successful weight loss program involves changes in behavior. Arguably, behavioral changes may be the most important part of a successful long-term weight loss program. The Weight Watchers program identifies two components of behavior that affect a dieter's success. These include self-monitoring and the thought process behind food choices. By addressing these two pieces of behavior, many hurdles previously thought to be insurmountable suddenly are approachable and attainable.

Barriers to Weight Loss

Binge Eating Disorder

Overweight and obesity are not the only manifestation of eating problems that affect fatty liver disease. Many different emotional disorders can promote weight gain or obstruct weight loss. Often, treatment of underlying conditions, such as depression, anxiety, or low self-esteem, should be concurrently initiated for weight loss to be successful. If you have a suspected emotional or psychiatric disorder, a referral for further evaluation and treatment is strongly advised prior to embarking on a weight management plan.

A wide range of disordered eating practices may be present in a person who is struggling to lose weight. These eating disorders, otherwise known as disordered eating, may

Case History

Ellen Grey

Ellen is 55 years old and was diagnosed with depression about 20 years ago. It was suggested that she start medications that would help with improving her mood. She took an antidepressant medication popular at that time, and noticed that her sleep improved considerably. In fact, the response was so great that she went off her medications a year later. About 5 years ago, Ellen started feeling fatigued. She had lost interest in the things that she normally liked to do. In fact, her husband noted that she rarely had the energy or desire to go out for walks or to the movies, both of which had been great sources of pleasure for her previously. She had increasing difficulty sleeping at night and constantly felt anxious. These symptoms were reminiscent of her major depressive episode 20 years prior. During the past 5 years, Ellen's weight steadily increased. She admitted that food was her only source of comfort, and that food was her only savior from spiraling deeper into oblivion. Consequently, her weight steadily increased, culminating in a 40-pound (18 kg) weight gain in this period of time. During her last check-up, Ellen's weight was 180 pounds (82 kg) with a BMI of 34. Her liver tests were all elevated, and she was newly diagnosed with diabetes.

Ellen's doctor recommended that she see a psychiatrist for a formal evaluation and in the interim started her on a new antidepressant medication. She was also told that a psychologist would be an excellent resource who could assist with behavioral therapy as needed. Within 8 weeks, her mood had improved considerably, along with her energy and sleeping patterns. She was advised not to come off her antidepressants unless there was a compelling need to do so, and then only under the supervision of her doctor. With her renewed zest for life, her eating patterns stabilized, as did her desire for reengaging with life, and within 6 months she had lost 25 pounds (11 kg), resulting in improved blood sugar and normalization of her liver tests.

range from simply skipping meals to full-blown binge eating disorders. A binge eating disorder is also called compulsive overeating. It is possibly the most common disordered eating behavior, present in 2% of all adults. Among mildly obese adults, between 10% and 15% of people will compulsively overeat, and among severely obese people, up to 40% will have disordered eating practices! People with a binge eating behavior typically consume large amounts of food and do not stop eating when they become full. They classically describe a feeling of loss of control and powerlessness to stop eating. This behavior may be triggered by stress, anxiety, guilt, or boredom.

Depression

Several medical studies have suggested a strong link between obesity and depression, especially in women, although it is unclear which of the two typically comes first. Patients with depression may present with a depressed or irritable mood and/ or a lack of interest in the daily activities of life. Interestingly, the diagnosis of depression may be challenging in obese patients, who can manifest their symptoms in turning to food for comfort to achieve some resolution of their mood. To ensure success, it is necessary to ensure that depression is treated appropriately prior to embarking on a plan for lifestyle modification, as both concentration and organization are required to cultivate new habits, and these traits may be compromised in a person who is still clinically depressed. If you feel signs of early depression, speak with your health-care professional for further guidance.

Causes of Binge Eating

The causes of binge eating are still unknown. Impulsive behavior may be more prevalent in people with binge eating disorder. Patients with binge eating disorder may gain and lose large amounts of weight rapidly. The weight loss is achieved through strict dieting. However, the pattern of overeating quickly resurfaces, resulting in rapid weight cycling. It is imperative that people with a binge eating disorder are not placed on a diet with less than 1400 to 1500 calories daily because very restrictive diets may worsen their binge eating pattern.

Diagnosis of Binge Eating Disorder

1. Eating much more rapidly than normal.
2. Eating until feeling uncomfortably full.
3. Eating large amounts of food when not feeling physically hungry.
4. Eating alone due to embarrassment at how much you are eating.
5. Feeling disgusted with yourself, depressed, or very guilty after overeating.
6. Marked distress about the binge eating behavior.

Diagnosis of Major Depression

1. Depressed mood most of the day.
2. Diminished interest or pleasure in all or almost all activities most of the day.
3. Significant weight gain or weight loss when not dieting.
4. Insomnia or increased hypersomnia nearly every day.
5. Agitation or lethargy nearly every day.
6. Feelings of worthlessness or excessive, inappropriate guilt.
7. Diminished ability to think or concentrate or indecisiveness.
8. Recurrent thoughts of death or self-harm.

Attention Deficit Disorder

Attention deficit disorder, with or without hyperactivity (ADD or ADHD) and impulsiveness, has been associated with increased risk for weight gain in both children and adults. One medical study confirmed that ADHD was present in more than 25% of all obese patients and 40% of patients with advanced obesity. Patients with ADD usually have a long history of impulsivity, lack of concentration, decreased attention, and inability to complete tasks. The need to diagnose this condition cannot be overstated; failure to do so will lead to lack of success with weight management strategies until impulsivity and lack of concentration are addressed.

Stress

Stress has both a psychological and physiological impact on weight management because it can affect a patient's eating and exercise behaviors. Stress induces a chemical response in the body that increases serum cortisol. Serum cortisol is a hormone that is produced in the adrenal gland and is responsible for regulating blood sugar levels and the immune system. It helps utilize fat and carbohydrate derived from the diet. Psychologically stressed individuals may find themselves more distracted, with decreased ability to focus, concentrate, and plan. People under stress may miss meals and snacks, thereby allowing extreme hunger to influence their eating decisions. Learning stress reduction methods and seeking professional assistance with management of stress will likely contribute toward better weight management. Meditation and deep-breathing exercises, along with aerobic exercise, are all excellent stress management techniques.

Case History (continued)

Karla

Karla has been following the Weight Watchers program for the past 16 weeks. She found that her weight loss has been slow and steady. She did not lose weight quickly in the early weeks of this diet plan, as she did with the Atkins diet. However, Karla has now lost 8 pounds (4 kg) in the past 16 weeks, and — surprisingly for her — she has been able to maintain that weight loss. She finds that she is still losing weight at a modest pace, but she does not feel deprived from treats or the occasional indulgence in comfort foods. She has been able to incorporate exercise into her regimen, and finds that her level of awareness about food and appropriate food choices has matured while on the Weight Watchers program.

CHAPTER 7

High-Fiber Foods and Prebiotics

Case History

Marvin Waters

Marvin is a 43-year-old male who has recently been diagnosed with NAFLD. He is known to have type 2 diabetes mellitus and is obese. He leads a relatively sedentary lifestyle due to his long hours at the office. He recently had a liver biopsy at the advice of his gastroenterologist, and the results showed moderately advanced disease consistent with inflammation and scarring, suggestive of NASH. He was told to make some fairly significant lifestyle changes or risk progression to full-blown cirrhosis. Marvin was quite concerned with these findings and with the possible progression of his disease. He had been doing some reading about prebiotic fibers and wanted further information with regard to the use of prebiotic fibers in NAFLD and NASH ...

(continued on page 85)

What is fiber? Fiber is probably best known for its ability to prevent or relieve constipation and to manage intestinal health. Although these functions of fiber are important for your health, there are myriad other health benefits attributable to fiber. Fiber can lower your risk of developing diabetes and heart disease, and it can help manage obesity and fatty liver disease. Dietary fiber, also known as roughage or bulk, includes all parts of plant foods that your body cannot digest or absorb. (Other food components, such as fats, proteins, and carbohydrates, can be broken down and absorbed in your intestine.) Fiber passes relatively intact through your stomach, small intestine, and colon, and then it moves into the rectum and out the anus as a bowel movement.

Kinds of Dietary Fiber

Dietary fiber comes in two forms: soluble and insoluble fiber. Soluble fibers predominate in oats, peas, peeled apples, citrus fruits, peeled carrots, and psyllium. The best sources of soluble fiber are dried beans and peas, oat products, and psyllium.

Soluble Fiber

Soluble fibers tend to hold on to water inside the small intestine and they thicken stool. Soluble fiber slows down the speed at which food travels through your gastrointestinal tract by increasing water absorption from the colon. This action encourages the formation of thickened, gel-like stools, and it lessens diarrhea. Soluble fibers help lower blood cholesterol and glucose levels. Dietary fiber is found mainly in fruits, vegetables, whole-grain products, and legumes.

Insoluble Fiber

Unlike soluble fiber, insoluble fiber does not dissolve in water. Insoluble fiber attracts fluid into the small intestine, resulting in the quicker movement of stool contents throughout the intestine, and it may improve symptoms of constipation. If a plant food appears rough in texture, is stringy, or has a tough skin or outer peel, it is most likely a source of insoluble fiber. Insoluble fibers are found in fruits and vegetables. Rich sources of insoluble fiber include whole wheat flour, wheat bran, nuts, and many vegetables, in particular the skins and seeds of vegetables.

> Insoluble fiber attracts fluid into the small intestine, resulting in the quicker movement of stool contents throughout the intestine.

Benefits of a High-Fiber Diet

1. *Normalizes bowel movements:* Dietary fiber increases the weight and size of your bowel movement, and it softens its texture. A bulky stool is easier to pass and reduces the risk of straining and pushing, thereby limiting the risk of developing hemorrhoids, which are potentially painful and may cause bleeding. Increased fiber intake also reduces the formation of diverticula in the bowel, which are pockets of weakness in the large intestine that may perforate, burst, or bleed, leading to severe abdominal pain and infection within the abdomen. Dietary fiber may also provide relief for people who suffer from diarrhea, because fiber can solidify stool by adding bulk and absorbing water.

2. *Lowers blood cholesterol levels and blood pressure:* The soluble fibers found in beans, oats, flax seeds, and oat bran may help lower total blood cholesterol levels by modulating the "bad" cholesterol levels. Medical studies have shown that increased fiber in the diet can also help reduce blood pressure, which is protective toward heart health. Aim to eat 10 grams of soluble fiber daily.

3. *Controls blood sugar levels:* Fiber, in particular soluble fiber, can slow the absorption of sugar from recently consumed food. This is great news for people who suffer from diabetes. Fiber has also been associated with preventing type 2 diabetes.

4. *Enables weight loss:* High-fiber foods are known to delay the movement of food and fluid through the stomach and intestine. This in part means that fiber-rich foods sit in your stomach slightly longer than other types of foods. When food is present in your stomach for a longer period of time, you experience a sense of fullness, or satiety, tricking your brain into believing that you are no longer hungry. Therefore, you stay satisfied or full for a greater period of time, reducing the amount of overall food and calories consumed. The risk of overeating is mitigated. Additionally, fiber-rich foods are generally less energy-dense. This means that fiber-rich foods have fewer calories — unit for unit — than many other foods, leading to more optimal weight control.

FAQ

Q. How much fiber should I eat?

A. The majority of people living in industrialized nations eat far too little fiber. The average North American consumes only 10 to 15 grams of fiber daily, but to achieve regularity in bowel movements and other health benefits, the target is between 25 and 30 grams of fiber daily. If you are currently not consuming much fiber and are keen on doing so, try and ramp up your fiber intake slowly. Incorporating 30 grams of fiber into your diet all at once runs you the risk of developing abdominal cramping, bloating, and perhaps some diarrhea. If you make the adjustment more gradually, your intestines will love you!

Q. Is fiber beneficial in fatty liver disease?

A. The most common risk factors for NAFLD include obesity and diabetes. By preventing these conditions, your risk of NAFLD decreases substantially. And, if already present, treating obesity and diabetes results in an improved course of liver disease and generally prevents progression to more advanced forms of disease. Robust fiber intake can improve the course of obesity and better modulate blood sugars, leading to the modification of risk factors and an improved course for fatty liver disease.

Good Sources of Insoluble Fiber

Food Item and Group	Serving Size	Fiber (grams)
Fresh and Dried Fruit		
Apple, with skin	1	2.6
Apricots, dried	¼ cup (60 mL)	2.9
Avocado	½	6.7
Banana	1	2.1
Blueberries	1 cup (250 mL)	4.0
Cherries	20	2.9
Figs, dried	¼ cup (60 mL)	3.7
Guava	1	4.9
Nectarine	1	2.4
Orange	1 large	3.3
Pear, with skin	1	5.0
Persimmon, Japanese	1	6.0
Prunes, dried and/or cooked	¼ cup (60 mL)	2.3–3.6
Strawberries	1 cup (250 mL)	3.4–3.9
Legumes, Pasta, Grain Products		
Black beans, boiled	1 cup (250 mL)	12.7
Bran cereal	1 cup (250 mL)	10.0–12.0
Bran flakes	1 cup (250 mL)	4.8
Bread (whole wheat, rye)	1 slice	3.0
Bulgur, cooked	1 cup (250 mL)	5.4
Corn bran, raw	¼ cup (60 mL)	15.8
Crackers, rye	3	7.5
English muffin (whole wheat)	1	4.4
Flax seeds (whole, ground)	1 tbsp (15 mL)	3.0
Hot multigrain cereal, cooked	¾ cup (175 mL)	4.0–5.1
Lentils, cooked	1 cup (250 mL)	8.9

Food Item and Group	Serving Size	Fiber (grams)
Muffin (oat bran)	1 small	3.0
Oat bran, cooked	¾ cup (175 mL)	2.1–3.3
Oats (rolled), cooked	1 cup (250 mL)	4.0
Pasta (whole wheat), cooked	1 cup (250 mL)	4.8
Quinoa, cooked	1 cup (250 mL)	4.1
Rice (brown, wild), cooked	1 cup (250 mL)	1.5–2.0
Rice bran, raw	¼ cup (60 mL)	4.2
Wheat bran, raw	¼ cup (60 mL)	11.4
Wheat germ, raw	¼ cup (60 mL)	3.5
Vegetables		
Artichoke, cooked	1	6.5
Broccoli, cooked	1 cup (250 mL)	4.0
Cabbage, cooked	1 cup (250 mL)	2.6
Carrot, cooked	1 cup (250 mL)	4.5
Cauliflower, cooked	1 cup (250 mL)	3.6–5.2
Corn (fresh or frozen), cooked	1 cup (250 mL)	3.4–4.4
Edamame, cooked	1 cup (250 mL)	8.6
Green peas, cooked	1 cup (250 mL)	7.4–11.2
Lima beans, cooked	1 cup (250 mL)	9.6
Potato (with skin), baked	1	2.8–4.3
Pumpkin (canned)	1 cup (250 mL)	7.6
Snap beans (green, yellow, Italian), cooked	1 cup (250 mL)	3.2
Spinach, cooked	1 cup (250 mL)	2.3–4.6
Squash (acorn, butternut), cooked	1 cup (250 mL)	3.6–4.2
Supplements		
Metamucil	1 tbsp (15 mL)	3.4
Psyllium husks, ground	1 tbsp (15 mL)	3.5

Good Sources of Soluble Fiber

Food Item and Group	Serving Size	Soluble Fiber (grams)
Fruits and Vegetables		
Asparagus, cooked	½ cup (125 mL)	1.7
Avocado	½	2.1
Brussels sprouts, cooked	½ cup (125 mL)	2.0
Edamame, cooked	½ cup (125 mL)	1.5
Figs, dried	¼ cup (60 mL)	1.9
Orange	1	1.8
Passion fruit	½ cup (125 mL)	6.5
Sweet potato (peeled), cooked	½ cup (125 mL)	1.8
Turnip, cooked	½ cup (125 mL)	1.7
Grain Products		
Bran buds with psyllium	⅓ cup (75 mL)	2.7
Oat bran, cooked	¾ cup (175 mL)	2.2
Oat flakes	1 cup (250 mL)	1.5
Legumes (Meat Alternatives)		
Beans, canned, with pork and tomato sauce	¾ cup (175 mL)	2.6
Black beans, cooked	¾ cup (175 mL)	5.4
Chickpeas, cooked	¾ cup (175 mL)	2.1
Kidney beans, cooked	¾ cup (175 mL)	2.6–3.0
Lima beans, cooked	¾ cup (175 mL)	5.3
Navy beans, cooked	¾ cup (175 mL)	3.3
Pinto beans, cooked	¾ cup (175 mL)	3.2
Soy burger	1 patty (85 g)	2.0
Soy nuts, roasted	¼ cup (60 mL)	3.5
Tofu, fried	¾ cup (175 mL)	2.8

Prebiotic Fiber

Prebiotic fiber can be found in health food stores and grocery stores in the form of powders, pills, or capsules. It is also added to common foods, such as yogurt and buttermilk. Prebiotics are thought to be beneficial to health.

Prebiotic fiber differs from other sources of fiber in that it has been proven in medical studies to alter the composition of gut bacteria in a favorable manner. Although both insoluble and soluble fibers have many beneficial properties, not all fibers impact the gut bacteria in the same manner.

Top 10 Food Sources of Prebiotics

Food	Prebiotic Fiber Content of Total Weight
Chicory root, raw	65%
Jerusalem artichoke, raw	32%
Dandelion greens, raw	24%
Garlic, raw	18%
Leek, raw	12%
Onion, raw / onion, cooked	9% / 5%
Asparagus, raw	5%
Wheat bran	5%
Whole wheat flour	5%
Banana, raw	1%

Functional Foods

Prebiotics are sometimes referred to as functional foods. A functional food is a cross between a food and a drug. In most countries, a prebiotic is accepted as a naturally occurring food substance that exerts many benefits seen otherwise through prescription medication use only.

- Prebiotics improve blood sugar control, regulate the metabolism of fats, and modify the bacteria that live in the gut. The gut is filled with billions of bacteria, all of which work synergistically to maintain human health. An imbalance between the "good" and "bad" bacteria in the gut can predispose an individual toward certain disease conditions.

- Prebiotics stimulate the growth of beneficial bacteria in the gut. In particular, bifidobacterium and lactobacillus are two types of bacteria that are known to have some very favorable effects on human health. These bacteria exert beneficial effects by lowering the acidity in the gastrointestinal tract, thereby impeding the growth of bacteria that are known to predispose toward illness and disease. The ability of some prebiotic-containing foods, such as Jerusalem artichokes and chicory, to modulate and regulate gut bacteria has been well established.

Prebiotics and Obesity

There is emerging evidence that the bugs in the gut can predispose toward obesity. When certain bugs are represented disproportionately in the gut, and other bugs are underrepresented, the balance may tip toward fat deposition. This is a whole area of medical research that is currently under investigation with regard to some of the mechanisms that lead toward obesity and NAFLD.

Because the impact of NAFLD on the liver is almost identical to the impact of alcohol, many researchers have questioned whether or not obesity predisposes toward alcohol production in the guts of people who do not consume alcohol. In fact, there have been some case reports of people who appear intoxicated but have not drunk a drop of alcohol! It is believed that these people may harbor intestinal bugs that produce large quantities of alcohol, causing the same effects as drinking extraneous sources. Although these case reports are exceedingly rare, it does raise an interesting question regarding the mechanisms that could potentially be contributing toward NAFLD. And — perhaps more importantly — it provides doctors and researchers with targets to study on the subject of specific treatment options, prebiotic fibers being one of these treatments.

Health Benefits of Prebiotic Fibers

- Improvement in blood sugar control
- Modest weight loss
- Improvement in blood cholesterol and triglyceride levels
- Improvement in liver enzymes
- Improvement in immune function
- Possible cancer-fighting properties

Benefits of Prebiotic Fibers

1. Reduces Production of Liver Fat

In addition to modifying the bacteria that reside in the gut, there is ample medical evidence that shows that prebiotic fibers reduce the liver's ability to produce fat. In part, NAFLD stems from excess fat deposited in the liver. That fat can come from excess fat consumed in the diet or from fat that is innately synthesized in the liver. In healthy people without NAFLD, the amount of fat that is naturally synthesized in the liver is relatively low. However, in people with NAFLD that natural synthesis of fat escalates. Prebiotic-rich diets may ameliorate NAFLD by reducing the amount of fat synthesized by the liver. It is believed that this is mediated by altering the genes that regulate fat metabolism.

2. Improves Obesity and Blood Sugar Control

People who have participated in studies of prebiotics have been asked to keep detailed records of food consumed. They found that energy intake was reduced in those who were taking prebiotic supplements — even though there was no active effort made to limit intake or to increase physical activity. Additionally, there were modest improvements in blood sugar control, and better regulation of a variety of hormones that have been known to influence appetite. Therefore, prebiotics are known to influence many of the risk factors that predispose toward NAFLD.

3. Improves Course of NAFLD

There have been very few studies that evaluated what happens to the liver of patients with NAFLD after consuming prebiotics for a period of time. Of the studies that are available, there appears to be a significant improvement in the liver tests among people who have supplemented with prebiotic fibers. However, none of the patients in any of these studies submitted to a liver biopsy to confirm definite improvement. Nonetheless, with the positive impact on risk factors for NAFLD, and the suggestion of improvement of liver tests, it seems reasonable to extrapolate the beneficial effects of prebiotic fibers on NAFLD.

Prebiotic Fiber Safety

The average daily intake of prebiotic fibers in the United States lies between 3 and 11 grams. Recently, prebiotic fibers have been added as ingredients to many common food products, notably in bread, cereal bars, and ready-to-eat breakfast cereals. Prebiotics are recognized as safe natural food ingredients in most countries.

Given that some of the prebiotic fibers are insoluble fibers, there may be some side effects, such as bloating, gas, and abdominal cramping, if used in particularly high doses. Therefore, prebiotic intake should be used judiciously in people who are predisposed toward these symptoms, such as those who suffer from irritable bowel syndrome.

Case History (continued)

Marvin

Marvin revisited his gastroenterologist's office for further discussion and counseling about his disease. He was reminded that modest weight loss primarily achieved through calorie restriction was the mainstay of therapy for his liver disease, and that modest exercise and physical activity would help immensely. However, Marvin was educated about the many benefits of prebiotic fibers and was encouraged to enrich his diet with prebiotic-containing foods and to aim to ingest between 20 and 30 grams of fiber daily.

Liver Detoxification

Fiber is also used to cleanse or detoxify the liver and the colon. There are many products available at your local pharmacy and health food store that claim to cleanse or flush toxins that may accumulate in your liver. None of these remedies has been proven in scientific studies to achieve this effect. Indeed, there are several undesirable side effects from using popular liver cleanses. Any detoxification program that involves rapid amounts of weight loss in a short period of time should be avoided.

Cleansing Tips

Without resorting to patent medicine to cleanse or detoxify your liver, you can adjust your eating and drinking habits to improve the overall quality of your health if you have fatty liver disease.

1. Keep yourself well hydrated. Most people do not drink enough water for the liver to function optimally. Drink 6 to 8 glasses of water every day. This should "wash" toxins through the liver to the kidneys to be expelled. Water is best. Most all other fluids have sugars or added chemicals that impede blood sugar control and predispose toward gastrointestinal complaints, such as diarrhea, bloating, and gas.

2. Eat lots of high-fiber, colorful foods, primarily fruit and vegetables, that are free of pesticides and other contaminants. Colorful fruit and vegetables are excellent sources of fiber, vitamins, and minerals that invigorate the liver and provide antioxidants to help repel disease. Given the high sugar content found in fruit, limit your fruit to 2 servings per day, but there is no limit on the amount of dark green leafy vegetables, broccoli, red tomatoes, yellow and red peppers, and beets that you can eat!

3. Try to cook with prebiotic fibers. A diet rich in prebiotic fibers may provide many beneficial effects, including modest amounts of weight loss, better control of your blood sugars, and reduced risks of heart disease.

4. Engage in a structured exercise program. Find an activity you truly enjoy that gets your blood pumping through your liver to be cleansed. Find something that rejuvenates you and makes you feel alive and youthful.

CHAPTER 8
Dietary Fats

Case History

Tony Toniel

Tony is 41 years old with a strong family history of heart disease. His father passed away from a heart attack at the age of 50, and his mother at the age of 55. Tony has been trying to quit smoking for the past 5 years, albeit unsuccessfully. He still smokes a pack daily, despite knowing that smoking is a major risk factor for heart disease. Recently, Tony found out he has fatty liver disease. He was told that NAFLD was a risk factor for heart disease. This gave Tony great concern for his health, resulting in greater attention to his dietary habits. He noted that there were many TV commercials talking about the fats in foods. In particular, he heard that trans fats were not good and increased the risk of dying from heart disease. He also heard that all fats had the same number of calories regardless of the fat source eaten. Tony was quite confused about the types of fats and was referred to a dietitian for further discussion ...

(continued page 103)

What are fats? There are three major kinds of dietary fats in the foods we eat. These include saturated fats, trans fats, and unsaturated fats, which include monounsaturated fat and polyunsaturated fat. These three types of fats have different chemical structures and properties. Saturated and trans fats tend to be more solid at room temperature, while monounsaturated and polyunsaturated fats tend to be more liquid at room temperature.

FAQ

Q. Which fats should I avoid? Are any fats good for me?

A. Trans fats should be avoided, and saturated fats should be limited. Fats affect the cholesterol levels in the body. The saturated and trans fats raise "bad" cholesterol levels in your blood. Monounsaturated fats may decrease the total cholesterol as well as the bad cholesterol. Polyunsaturated fats can not only decrease the total cholesterol (including the bad cholesterol), but certain types of polyunsaturated fats may also protect against heart disease and sudden death. And they have beneficial effects on the nervous system too.

Kinds of Fat

Saturated fats

Unsaturated fats
Monounsaturated fats
Polyunsaturated fats

Trans fats

Omega-3 essential fatty acids
Alpha-linolenic acid (ALA)
Docosahexaenoic acid (DHA)
Eicosapentaenoic acid (EPA)

Omega-6 essential fatty acids

Macronutrient Calories

Macronutrient	Calories Per Gram Consumed
Carbohydrate	4
Fat	9
Protein	4

Saturated Fats

Many foods contain both saturated and unsaturated fats, but a particular food item is generally described by the type of fat that predominates. Saturated fats occur naturally in many foods. They are needed for the production of hormones, the stabilization of cellular membranes, the padding around organs, and energy. A deficiency in the consumption of saturated fats can lead to dysfunction of the immune system, resulting in increased vulnerability to infection.

The majority of saturated fats come from animal sources, including meat and dairy products. Examples include fatty beef, lamb, pork, poultry, lard, cream, and butter. For this reason, many baked goods and fried foods contain high levels of saturated fats.

To avoid increasing your risk of heart disease, high cholesterol, and stroke, it's best to minimize your intake of saturated fats to 7% of your daily total energy intake. For example, if you require 2000 calories daily, do not consume more than 140 calories, or 16 grams, from saturated fat sources.

Sources of Saturated Fats

The amounts of saturated fat and total fat in this table are per 100 grams of edible food portion.

Fat Source	Saturated Fat	Total Fat
Beef, ground, 75% lean meat, 25% fat, patty, broiled	6.77 g	17.82 g
Beef, top sirloin, trimmed, lean only, cooked, broiled	2.22 g	5.84 g
Cheese, Cheddar	21.09 g	33.16 g
Cheese, cottage (low-fat, 1% milk fat)	0.65 g	1.02 g
Cheese, cream	21.97 g	34.90 g
Cheese, Swiss	17.78 g	27.80 g
Chicken broilers or fryers, wing, meat with skin, cooked, fried with batter	5.83 g	21.82 g
Chicken broilers, skinless, white meat only	1.01 g	3.57 g
Chicken pot pie, frozen entrée	4.45 g	13.41 g
Cream, heavy or whipping (35%)	23.03 g	37.00 g
Cream, whipped cream topping, pressurized	13.83 g	22.33 g
Milk, canned, sweetened condensed	5.49 g	8.70 g
Milk, low-fat, 1% milk fat	0.63 g	0.97 g
Milk, whole, 3.25% milk fat	1.87 g	3.25 g
Pork (including bacon), cured, cooked, broiled, pan-fried, roasted	13.74 g	41.79 g
Pork (including spareribs), fresh, separable lean and fat, cooked, braised	11.12 g	30.31 g

Recommendations by the American Dietetic Association and Dietitians of Canada

for total fat (for adults) and saturated, monounsaturated, and polyunsaturated fatty acids based on a 2000-calorie diet

Total Fat	Amount (grams)
20% of energy	44
25% of energy	56
30% of energy	67
35% of energy	78
Saturated Fatty Acid (SFA) (not to exceed 7% of total daily energy)	
3% of energy	7
7% of energy	16
10% of energy	22
Monounsaturated Fatty Acid	
8% of energy	18
14% of energy	31
20% of energy	44
25% of energy	56
Polyunsaturated (Omega-6) Fatty Acid (3% to 10% of energy)	

Trans Fats

Trans fats are created in an industrial process that adds hydrogen to liquid vegetable oils to make them more solid. Another term used to describe these is "partially hydrogenated oils." Food companies like to use trans fats because they are inexpensive to produce and last a long time. Additionally, trans fats give foods a rich taste and texture. Many restaurants and fast-food joints use trans fats to deep-fry foods, because oils with trans fats can be used repeatedly in commercial fryers.

Trans fats are the undesirable fats. Trans fats raise your bad cholesterol (LDL) and lower your good cholesterol (HDL) levels. Trans fats are also associated with developing type 2 diabetes. All of these conditions increase your risk of death from heart disease, in addition to increasing your risk for liver disease from NAFLD. Trans fats can be found in many foods, but most notably in french fries, shortenings, doughnuts, and baked goods, such as pastries, piecrusts, pizza dough, cookies, and crackers. By reading food labels, you can identify the presence of trans fats.

Common Sources of Trans Fats

Food	Trans Fats in a Single Serving (grams)
Microwave popcorn	6
Beef pot pie (from frozen)	2
Blueberry muffin mix	1.5
Crescent rolls, refrigerated	1.5
Cake mix	0.5
Frozen chicken and noodles dinner	0.5

How to Minimize Your Risk from Eating Trans Fats

1. Follow the suggestions in Health Canada's Eating Well with Canada's Food Guide or the Federal Department of Agriculture (FDA) Choose MyPlate guide, which advise you to lower your intake of dairy products, eat leaner meats, and try preparing foods with little or no fat.
2. Read the labels on packaged food products. Since December 2005, in Canada, it is usually mandatory to list the amount of trans fat on the food label. Also, look for the term "partially hydrogenated oil." If you see this phrase on the label, it means that the product contains trans fat.
3. Choose soft margarines that are labeled "free of trans fat" or "made with non-hydrogenated fat."
4. Minimize consumption of fried foods. When you do fry foods, use healthier oils that contain a higher proportion of monounsaturated fats.
5. When you eat out, ask your server about the trans fat content of the foods on the menu. Some restaurants have a "nutritional content" list on their website or will provide one if requested.

DID YOU KNOW?

Trans Fat Limits
The American Heart Association recommends that adults limit their consumption of trans fats to less than 1% of total energy daily. In other words, if you require 2000 calories daily, no more than 20 calories, or less than 2 grams of your food intake, should come from trans fats sources. Unlike the other sources of fat, trans fats have no essential human function and are not required for human health.

Unsaturated Fats

Unsaturated fats are considered to be good fats. There are two types of unsaturated fats: monounsaturated and polyunsaturated fats. Monounsaturated and polyunsaturated fats differ in their chemical structure. Monounsaturated fats are simply fats that have one double bond carbon in the molecule; polyunsaturated fats have more than one double bond carbon in their chemical structure. The fats in the food you eat should not exceed more than 25% to 35% of the total calories you eat daily. The majority of the fats you consume should be in the form of monounsaturated or polyunsaturated fats.

Monounsaturated Fats

Monounsaturated fats are typically liquid at room temperature but start to turn solid when chilled. Olive oil is the classic monounsaturated fat.

When consumed in moderation, monounsaturated fats have a beneficial effect on health by reducing bad cholesterol and lowering the risk of heart disease and stroke. Vegetable oils, including olive oil, canola oil, peanut oil, sunflower oil, and sesame oil, are rich in monounsaturated fats. Other sources include avocados, peanut butter, and many nuts and seeds.

Polyunsaturated Fats

Polyunsaturated fats are one of the major types of unsaturated fats with beneficial properties for health. In moderation, polyunsaturated fats help reduce cholesterol levels and lower risk of heart disease and premature death. They include the essential fats that your body needs but cannot synthesize by itself, and they must be obtained from food sources — such as a number of vegetable oils, including soybean oil, corn oil, and safflower oil, in addition to fatty fish, including salmon, mackerel, herring, and trout. These essential fats include the omega-3 and omega-6 series of essential fatty acids (EFAs).

Essential Fatty Acids

Rich in polyunsaturated fat, there are two series of essential fats, omega-3 and omega-6 fats, and they impact health differently.

Omega-3 Essential Fatty Acids

FAQ

Q. **What are omega-3 fatty acids?**

A. Omega-3 fatty acids are polyunsaturated fatty acids. Omega-3 fatty acids are considered essential fatty acids. This means that they need to be obtained from your diet because they are not produced by your body. Omega-3 fatty acids are essential to many of the functions of the body. Omega-3 fatty acids assist with blood clotting and with building cell membranes in the brain.

There are three types of omega-3 fatty acids:
- Alpha-linolenic acid (ALA)
- Docosahexaenoic acid (DHA)
- Eicosapentaenoic acid (EPA)

Omega-3 Fatty Acid Conversion

Alpha-linolenic acid (ALA) is the most common type of omega-3 fatty acid, found in some vegetable oils, such as soybean, rapeseed (canola), and flaxseed. ALA is also found in some green vegetables, such as Brussels sprouts, kale, spinach, and salad greens. ALA is considered the "parent" in the omega-3 family and can be converted into the other omega-3 fats: docosahexaenoic acid (DHA) and eicosapentaenoic acid (EPA). The conversion of ALA to EPA and DHA is limited. Only about 1% of ALA is converted in the body to EPA and DHA — not enough to meet your dietary needs, making it necessary to supplement or fortify the diet with plant and fish oils. Some processed foods are fortified with omega-3 fatty acids, but the doses are generally quite low, and supplementation is still needed for good health.

Good Sources of Omega-3 Fatty Acids Rich in EPA and DHA	Grams of Omega-3 Fatty Acid per 3-oz (90 g) Serving
Cod	0.15–0.24
Flounder	0.48
Halibut	0.60-–1.12
Herring, sardines	1.30–2.00
Mackerel	1.10–1.70
Red snapper	0.29

Good Sources of Omega-3 Fatty Acids Rich in EPA and DHA	Grams of Omega-3 Fatty Acid per 3-oz (90 g) Serving
Salmon	1.10–1.90
Tuna (fresh)	0.21–1.10
Tuna (canned)	0.17–0.24

Health Benefits of Omega-3 Fatty Acids

Fatty liver management: The latest medical evidence suggests that increased dietary intake of omega-3 fatty acids from fish-based sources benefits people with fatty liver disease. Omega-3 fats favorably affect blood pressure and triglyceride levels, which are major risks for NAFLD. By altering these risks, the progression of NAFLD may be curtailed. In addition to these effects, the benefits of EPA and DHA include the ability to alter the genes in the liver that metabolize fat. Instead of fat synthesis and storage in the liver, omega-3 fats contribute toward utilization of the liver fat, so that fat storage in the liver is minimized. Additionally, omega-3 fats improve insulin function. The anti-inflammatory properties of omega-3 fats reduce liver inflammation, thereby leading to improved liver biopsy results.

Cardiovascular management: Two omega-3 fatty acids, DHA and EPA, have been associated with cardiovascular benefit. The most compelling evidence for the cardiac benefits provided by omega-3 fats comes from three extremely large medical trials that showed reductions in heart events, ranging between 20% and 0%! These findings strongly suggest that omega-3 fat consumption, whether from dietary sources or supplements in the form of fish oil, should be increased, especially in those patients with or at risk for coronary artery disease. Emerging evidence has not confirmed these effects from supplement use, leading researchers to wonder whether previously observed beneficial cardiac effects were limited to consumption of fresh fish alone.

Lipid management: Additionally, studies confirm that a diet rich in omega-3 fatty acids may help lower triglycerides and increase HDL ("good") cholesterol. Omega-3 fatty acids may thin the blood when consumed in larger doses, protecting against the development of coronary heart disease.

Inflammation management: Omega-3 fatty acids possess anti-inflammatory, anti-arrhythmic, and anticlotting properties. Many disease states that are driven and mediated by inflammation appear to be favorably impacted by the consistent use of omega-3 fatty acids.

Blood pressure management: Other studies have confirmed that omega-3 fats lower blood pressure in those who suffer from high blood pressure. Collectively, the positive impact of omega-3 fats on triglycerides, blood pressure, and heart disease cannot be ignored.

FAQ

Q. How much omega-3 fatty acid should I consume?

A. At this time, there is not that much evidence in the literature to guide the dosage of omega-3 fats with the goal of inducing success in NAFLD; however, a rough guideline based on the existing literature would range between 1 and 3 grams of EPA and DHA daily.

People with known coronary heart disease or risk factors for the same should aim to consume 1 gram of EPA and DHA daily. The doses necessary to modify triglyceride levels, however, are much higher: approximately 3 to 4 grams of EPA and DHA daily. At these doses, research shows that triglyceride levels are lowered by 20% to 50%. Oral supplements from a health food store or drug store are not necessarily more favorable than the intake of fish. The best strategy may be to eat more fish.

Q. Are there any side effects associated with omega-3 fatty acids?

A. The majority of side effects arising from omega-3 fatty acid intake occur in the context of omega-3 supplements, not omega-3-rich foods. Omega-3 fatty acids are generally safe and do not cause serious side effects. There is a theoretical risk of abnormal bleeding as a result of fish oil consumption at higher doses, but this has seldom manifested as a real cause for concern, and, generally, it is not recommended to limit fish oil consumption due to this concern. Another theoretical concern is an increase in LDL ("bad") cholesterol with high doses of fish oil, but again, the relevance of this theoretical abnormality is unclear, and restriction of fish oil due to this concern is unwarranted unless very high doses of omega-3 fats are used. More common side effects include a fishy aftertaste and loose bowel movements.

Mercury Poisoning Risk

There is a concern for high mercury intake and potential mercury poisoning in diets rich in certain types of fish. High-mercury fish include shark, swordfish, and tuna (fresh, frozen, and canned white tuna). Low-mercury fish include canned light tuna, salmon, sardines, anchovies, cod, crab, haddock, halibut, pollack, sole, trout, and shrimp. Typically, only pregnant women, women contemplating pregnancy, women who are breastfeeding, and young children are encouraged to avoid eating some types of fish due to this risk. High-quality fish oil supplements usually do not contain this contaminant.

American Heart Association Recommendations for Omega-3 Fatty Acid Intake

Patient Population	Recommendation
Patients with no documented history of coronary heart disease	Eat a variety of fish (preferably oily fish) at least twice weekly. Include oils and foods rich in alpha-linolenic acid (flaxseed, canola, and soybean oils; walnuts).
Patients with documented history of coronary artery disease	Consume approximately 1 gram of EPA plus DHA daily, preferably from oily fish. EPA plus DHA capsule supplements may be used in consultation with a physician.
Patients who need to lower triglyceride level	Consume 2 to 4 grams of EPA plus DHA in capsule supplement form, in consultation with a physician.

Omega-3 Fatty Acid Review
Benefits of Omega-3 Essential Fatty Acids

1. Reduces risk for sudden death.
2. Reduces death from all causes.
3. Lowers blood triglyceride levels.
4. Provides modest effect on lowering blood pressure in patients with known high blood pressure.
5. Shows beneficial effects on the liver in patients with NAFLD.
6. Reduces morning stiffness and decreases the number of tender swollen joints in patients with rheumatoid arthritis.

Side Effects

1. Generally well tolerated.
2. Fishy aftertaste.
3. Nausea, bloating, belching at times.

4. Theoretical increased risk of bleeding (not deemed to be significant).
5. Theoretical increased risk of LDL ("bad") cholesterol when used at higher doses.
6. Environmental exposure to contaminants with certain fish species.

Dosage and Safety

Capsules: A 1-gram capsule generally contains about 180 mg of EPA and 120 mg of DHA

Interactions: No significant drug interactions

For cardiac health: Approximately 1 gram of EPA plus DHA daily

For lowering triglycerides: 2 to 4 grams of EPA plus DHA daily

For NAFLD: It's not yet clearly defined, but the range is between 1 and 3 grams of EPA plus DHA daily

Omega-6 Essential Fatty Acids

Omega-6 fatty acids are essential fatty acids similar to omega-3 fatty acids. Again, this means that they must be obtained from the diet because the body does not naturally synthesize them. Omega-6 fatty acids have health benefits involving brain function, maintenance of bone health, and regulation and maintenance of the reproductive system. They are also required for normal growth and development.

Excess Omega-6 EFAs

Diets rich in omega-6 fatty acids may lead to increased risks of heart disease, arthritis, and possibly cancer. Excess omega-6 intake interferes with the health benefits of omega-3 fats in part because they compete for the same enzymes, resulting in the decreased formation of omega-3 metabolites. Routine supplementation of omega-6 fatty acids is generally not recommended because most people ingest large quantities of omega-6 fatty acids in their regular diet. If you are interested in supplementing with omega-6 fatty acids, you should have a discussion with your health-care professional.

How to Increase Omega-3 to Omega-6 Ratio

1. *Change your cooking oil.* Vegetable oils that contain large amounts of omega-6 fatty acids and low amounts of omega-3 should be avoided. The top offenders are grape-seed, cottonseed, safflower, corn, and sunflower oils. Alternatives are olive, macadamia, avocado, and canola oils.

DID YOU KNOW?

Omega-3 to Omega-6 Ratio

A healthy diet contains a balance between omega-3 and omega-6 fats. However, most Westerners consume too many omega-6 fatty acids. Although omega-3 fatty acids are known to exert anti-inflammatory effects, omega-6 fatty acids tend to promote inflammation. Other negative effects of consuming excess omega-6 fatty acids include the promotion of clotting and the constriction, or tightening, of blood vessels. The typical American diet tends to contain 15 to 20 times more omega-6 fatty acids than omega-3 fatty acids — in contrast to the Mediterranean diet, which has a healthier balance between omega-3 and omega-6 fats.

2. *Limit processed foods.* This is one of the best methods to cut down on omega-6 fats. If you choose whole foods over processed ones, you can probably slash over one-third of omega-6 fats from your diet.
3. *Read food labels.* This is a valuable tip not just for recognizing high omega-6 foods, but also for most other nutritional information as well, including sodium, protein, and other ingredients.

Good Sources of Omega-6 Fatty Acids

Seeds and nuts are rich in omega-6 fatty acids. Processed snack foods are usually high in omega-6 content. This is primarily due to the vegetable oils that are included in most commercial American snack foods. Fast foods also tend to be high in omega-6 fatty acids. A typical fish sandwich provides about 8 grams, a fast-food chicken sandwich contains 10 grams, and a hamburger dressed with the standard toppings contains 7 grams. Meats are a rich source of omega-6 fats too, with the number dependent on the cooking style. A batter-fried chicken provides 38 grams of omega-6 fatty acids, but a stewed chicken contains only 17 grams.

Foods Rich in Omega-6 Fatty Acids

Food	Serving Size	Amount
Oils		
Safflower oil (70% linoleic)	1 tbsp (15 mL) = 13.8 g	10.3 g
Vegetable oil, canola and soybean	1 tbsp (15 mL) = 13.8 g	3.2 g
Vegetable oil, corn	1 tbsp (15 mL) = 13.8 g	7.4 g
Vegetable oil, corn and canola	1 tbsp (15 mL) = 14.2 g	3.3 g
Vegetable oil, corn, peanut and olive	1 tbsp (15 mL) = 13.8 g	4.5 g
Vegetable oil, cottonseed	1 tbsp (15 mL) = 13.8 g	7.1 g
Vegetable oil, grapeseed	1 tbsp (15 mL) = 13.8 g	9.6 g
Vegetable oil, sesame	1 tbsp (15 mL) = 13.8 g	5.7 g
Vegetable oil, soybean	1 tbsp (15 mL) = 13.8 g	7.0 g
Vegetable oil, soybean lecithin	1 tbsp (15 mL) = 13.8 g	5.5 g

Food	Serving Size	Amount
Vegetable oil, sunflower, linoleic (60% and over)	1 tbsp (15 mL) = 13.8 g	9.1 g
Vegetable oil, sunflower, linoleic (less than 60%)	1 tbsp (15 mL) = 13.8 g	5.5 g
Vegetable oil, walnut	1 tbsp (15 mL) = 13.8 g	7.3 g
Vegetable oil, wheat germ	1 tbsp (15 mL) = 13.8 g	7.6 g
Nuts		
Almonds, dried, blanched (slices)	¼ cup (60 mL) = 241 g	2.9 g
Almonds, dried, blanched (whole)	¼ cup (60 mL) = 36.8 g	4.4 g
Almonds, dry-roasted, not blanched (whole)	¼ cup (60 mL) = 35.0 g	4.4 g
Almonds, honey-roasted, not blanched (whole)	¼ cup (60 mL) = 36.5 g	3.7 g
Almonds, oil-roasted, blanched (whole)	¼ cup (60 mL) = 36.0 g	4.1 g
Almonds, oil-roasted, not blanched (whole)	¼ cup (60 mL) = 39.8 g	5.4 g
Almonds, toasted, not blanched	¼ cup (60 mL) = 35.0 g	3.6 g
Brazil nuts, dried, not blanched	¼ cup (60 mL) = 35.5 g	7.3 g
Butternuts (white walnuts), dried	¼ cup (60 mL) = 30.4 g	10.3 g
Cashew butter, plain	2 tbsp (30 mL) = 32.4 g	2.6 g
Cashew nuts, dry-roasted (whole or halves)	¼ cup (60 mL) = 34.7 g	2.7 g
Cashew nuts, oil-roasted (whole or halves)	¼ cup (60 mL) = 32.7 g	2.8 g
Cashew nuts, raw	¼ cup (60 mL) = 33.0 g	2.6 g
Pecans, dried (halves)	¼ cup (60 mL) = 25.1 g	5.2 g
Pecans, dry-roasted	¼ cup (60 mL) = 27.9 g	5.5 g

Food	Serving Size	Amount
Pecans, oil-roasted	¼ cup (60 mL) = 27.9 g	6.3 g
Pistachios, dry-roasted	¼ cup (60 mL) = 31.2 g	4.3 g
Pistachios, raw	¼ cup (60 mL) = 31.2 g	4.2 g
Walnuts, black, dried (chopped)	¼ cup (60 mL) = 31.7 g	10.5 g
Walnuts, English or Persian, dried (halves)	¼ cup (60 mL) = 25.4 g	9.7 g
Seeds		
Pumpkin seed kernels	¼ cup (60 mL)	10.0 g
Sesame seeds	¼ cup (60 mL)	7.5 g
Sunflower seed kernels, oil-roasted, salted	¼ cup (60 mL) = 34.2 g	34.1 g
Sunflower seed kernels, oil-roasted, unsalted	¼ cup (60 mL) = 34.2 g	11.7 g
Margarine		
Margarine, canola and safflower oils (non-hydrogenated), such as Becel	1 tbsp (15 mL) = 14.8 g	3.2 g
Margarine, soya oil (non-hydrogenated)	1 tbsp (15 mL) = 14.8 g	4.4 g
Other Foods		
Chicken, roasting, drumstick, meat and skin, roasted	1 drumstick (3 oz/90 g)	2.4 g
Egg (of chicken), whole, boiled in shell, hard-cooked	2 large	1.3 g
Peanut butter	¼ cup (60 mL)	10.0 g

Alpha-Linolenic Acid (ALA) Content of Various Foods and Oils

Nuts (per 100 grams raw edible portion)	ALA (grams)
Flax seeds	22.8
Butternuts (dried)	8.7
Walnuts	4.0–7.0
Chia seeds (dried)	3.9
Beechnuts (dried)	1.7
Almonds	0.4
Peanuts	0.003

Vegetables (per 100 grams raw edible portion)	ALA (grams)
Seaweed (spirulina)	0.8
Leeks (freeze-dried)	0.7
Kale	0.2
Lettuce	0.1
Spinach	0.1

Legumes (per 100 grams raw edible portion)	ALA (grams)
Soybeans (dry)	1.6
Beans (common, dry)	0.6
Cowpeas (dry)	0.3
Lima beans (dry)	0.2
Peas, garden (dry)	0.2

Grains	ALA (grams)
Oat germ	1.4
Wheat germ	0.7
Corn germ	0.3
Rice bran	0.2

Essential Fatty Acids in Common Oils

Omega-3 Fatty Acid Oils	Omega-6 Fatty Acid Oils
Fish oil	Borage oil
Flaxseed oil	Corn oil
Soybean oil	Cottonseed oil
Walnut oil	Peanut oil
	Primrose oil
	Safflower oil
	Sesame oil
	Soybean oil (higher than in omega-3)
	Sunflower oil

How to Choose Healthy Fats

1. Read the nutrition labels on packaged food and choose foods with lower fat content.
2. Limit your intake of saturated and trans fats. Choose soft margarines that are low in saturated and trans fat, or opt for a non-hydrogenated margarine. Substitute soft margarine for hard margarine, butter, or lard in baking.
3. Choose leaner cuts of meat. Opt for skinless chicken and turkey, or remove the skin before cooking to lower intake of saturated fats.
4. Eat fish at least two or three times weekly to increase your intake of omega-3 essential fatty acids.
5. Choose lower-fat dairy options to reduce your intake of saturated fats.
7. Buy fewer packaged foods and "ready to eat" meals to avoid trans fats.
8. Buy vegetables, fruits, and whole-grain products with no added fat.
9. Consider meat alternatives, such as beans, lentils, nuts, seeds, and tofu, to lower your intake of saturated fats.
10. Use vegetable oils, such as canola and olive oils. Use very small amounts of vegetable oils for stir-frying or sautéing. One teaspoon (5 mL) is usually sufficient.
11. Heat oil before frying to prevent food from soaking up the oil.

12. Fill a spray bottle with vegetable oil and spray the pan instead of greasing.
13. Make your own salad dressing with canola or olive oil. Add balsamic, rice wine, or other vinegars.
14. When eating out, ask for gravy, sauces, and dressings to be served on the side. Use only small amounts of these.
15. Ask your server for the nutritional breakdown of the menu items before you order. Some restaurants have this information posted on their website or have a pamphlet available in the kitchen.

Case History (continued)

Tony

We explained to Tony the key classes of fats, including saturated, trans fats, and unsaturated (monounsaturated and polyunsaturated) fats. He learned that all fats had 9 calories per gram, which made any source of fat energy-dense, and eating in excess of recommended fat amounts would lead to weight gain. However, that's where the similarity between the classes of fats ended. Saturated fats and trans fats increased the risk of high cholesterol and heart disease, whereas the unsaturated fats decreased this risk. Additionally, there were some beneficial properties of omega-3 fats, particularly in people at higher risk of developing heart disease, in those who already had heart disease, and in those with NAFLD. Tony found out that fats were essential for health, and learned what amounts of each type of fat he should be aiming to consume daily. Lastly, he learned about the sources of each type of fat, and some quick tips about minimizing the bad fats while maximizing the good fats.

CHAPTER 9

Nutritional Supplementation

Case History

Sandy Brown

Sandy is a 33-year-old overweight woman with a BMI of 28. She has high blood pressure and borderline high triglycerides. She was only recently diagnosed with NAFLD, although her liver enzymes have been elevated for a number of years. Sandy was recently speaking to one of her friends, who advised her of the benefits of omega-3 and omega-6 fatty acids. Sandy had always been open to more complementary therapies, and was quite interested in learning more about the possible role for omega-3 fatty acid supplements given her liver disease. She had questions surrounding their use, efficacy, dosage, and whether or not supplements were preferable to naturally occurring foods ...

(continued on page 109)

Besides vitamin E and essential fatty acids, several other micronutrients, in particular chromium and vitamin D, have shown a positive impact on fatty liver disease. Some of these micronutrients are available in food, although recommended amounts are sometimes difficult to achieve through diet alone and need to be supplemented.

Chromium

Chromium is an essential micronutrient that plays a role in how insulin helps the body regulate blood sugar levels. Insulin resistance is very common in fatty liver disease and is a prime feature in patients with type 2 diabetes. Many North Americans' diets are low in chromium. However, at present, there is no standard method to measure chromium levels in your system.

Best Food Sources of Chromium

Chromium is found in a variety of foods in small amounts. Choose whole wheat products to maximize the chromium in your diet.

Fruits and Vegetables	Meats	Grains
Broccoli	Beef	Whole wheat bagels
Grape juice	Ham	Whole wheat breads
Orange juice	Turkey	Whole wheat muffins

Supplement Dosage

There is a considerable array of chromium dosages available in supplement form. In medical studies that have evaluated the efficacy on diabetes, high doses ranging between 400 and 1000 mcg (micrograms) have been used safely, even though these doses exceed the adequate intake level set by scientific committees. We recommend diets rich in chromium rather than supplements for patients with diabetes or NAFLD.

Vitamin D

Vitamin D is a fat-soluble vitamin best known for its role in the absorption and metabolism of calcium, which is essential in maintaining healthy bones. Any fat-soluble vitamin requires appropriate digestion and absorption of fat from food. A disorder that compromises this function may contribute toward a deficiency of that particular vitamin.

Associated Functional Disorders

Cancer: Various studies have shown that people with adequate levels of vitamin D have a significantly lower risk of developing cancer compared to people with lower levels.

Immunity: Vitamin D regulates the immune system and contributes toward fighting inflammation and infection.

Multiple sclerosis: Vitamin D may also reduce the risk of developing multiple sclerosis. Multiple sclerosis is much less common in countries clustered in the equatorial regions, meaning that their populations are generally blessed with more hours of sunlight.

DID YOU KNOW?

Divided Opinion

There is some evidence to suggest that chromium supplements can help people with diabetes lower their blood sugar levels. Researchers have studied the effects of chromium supplements on diabetes for many years, but medical studies are divided with regard to the efficacy. Some studies have found no benefit, whereas other studies have reported that chromium supplements may reduce blood sugar levels.

Rickets: Inadequate vitamin D intake can predispose toward rickets, which is a disease that leads to the softening and weakening of bones. In some ways, rickets is similar to osteoporosis.

Vitamin D Sources

Vitamin D is obtained primarily from sunlight exposure. Food sources can provide relatively modest doses of vitamin D. People who are exposed to adequate amounts of sunlight are generally not at risk of vitamin D deficiency. Lack of vitamin D production in the skin may occur in people who live in climates with little exposure to sunlight. Canada, Norway, Sweden, Denmark, and Iceland are prime examples of these types of climates. There is limited daylight in these northern countries during the winter months, leading to vitamin D deficiency in this time period. During the summer months, however, there is adequate daylight exposure.

Even in countries with adequate daylight exposure, staying indoors without exposure to sunlight can lead to vitamin D deficiency. Covered arms and legs will preclude the body's ability to synthesize vitamin D. You may not get enough vitamin D from your diet if you are lactose intolerant and do not supplement with vitamin D. A vegetarian diet and one low in milk products are also risks for vitamin D deficiency.

Vitamin D and Fatty Liver Disease

One of the roles ascribed to vitamin D is the maintenance of a well-controlled immune system. In the liver, vitamin D may suppress the development of fibrosis, or scarring. There have been some animal studies that showed improvement in animals with NAFLD/NASH who were treated with exposure to light and vitamin D supplementation. There are some human studies, although limited, that show that people with low vitamin D levels are more likely to have NAFLD.

Vitamin D Check-up

It is not recommended to have vitamin D levels checked if you are relatively healthy and are without diseases that affect your absorptive capacity. Some examples of diseases and conditions that can affect the absorption of food and nutrients include Crohn's disease, celiac disease, diseases of the pancreas, and multiple surgeries involving the small intestine. Other conditions, such as diabetes, high blood pressure, and heart diseases, should not affect vitamin D levels. If you have NAFLD without inflammation or fibrosis, it is not necessary to have your vitamin D levels checked. However, you should focus on strategies to maximize your vitamin D levels. If you have NASH (NAFLD with inflammation and fibrosis), check your vitamin D levels, because higher dosing strategies may be required to correct the deficiency.

FAQ

Q. How do I know if I am vitamin D deficient?

A. The only way to truly know if you are vitamin D deficient is to check your blood levels for vitamin D, specifically 25-hydroxyvitamin D_3 (25OHD3) levels. Liver diseases that have advanced into cirrhosis can also predispose to vitamin D deficiency.

Q. How much vitamin D do I need?

A. For the majority of adults under 70 years of age, 600 international units (IUs) daily is the recommendation. The tolerable upper intake level is set as 4000 IUs daily. These levels are set for adults who experience very minimal sunlight exposure. For northern geographical climates, including the northern United States, Canada, and other countries with similar latitudes, if you are getting a reasonable amount of sunlight exposure during the summer months, a supplement is not necessary during this time. However, supplementing with 1000 IUs of vitamin D during the winter months is recommended. Darker-skinned individuals do not synthesize vitamin D as efficiently; therefore, supplementing year-round with 1000 IUs daily is recommended. The above suggestions are for individuals who have not had their vitamin D levels checked and are generally not at risk of having vitamin D deficiency from underlying medical problems. If you have a medical condition in which you do not absorb nutrients effectively, the recommendations for vitamin D repletion are different and it is important to consult with your physician before supplementing with vitamin D.

Food Sources of Vitamin D

Food	Serving Size	International Units (IUs) Per Serving
Cod liver oil	1 tbsp (15 mL)	1360
Salmon (sockeye), cooked	3 oz (90 g)	447
Tuna, canned in water	3 oz (90 g)	154
Orange juice fortified with vitamin D	1 cup (250 mL)	137
Milk fortified with vitamin D (nonfat, reduced fat, and whole)	1 cup (250 mL)	115–124
Yogurt fortified with vitamin D	6 oz (175 g)	80
Margarine fortified with vitamin D	1 tbsp (15 mL)	60
Sardines, canned in oil	2 sardines	46
Liver (beef), cooked	3 oz (90 g)	42
Egg (vitamin D is found in yolk)	1 large	41
Ready-to-eat cereal fortified with vitamin D	1 cup (250 mL) dry	40
Cheese, Swiss	1 oz (30 g)	6

FAQ

Q. **Am I at risk for vitamin D toxicity?**

A. Vitamin D toxicity is a rare but potentially serious condition that occurs when you have excessive amounts of vitamin D in your system. Vitamin D toxicity is usually caused by extremely large doses of vitamin D in supplement form; it is not caused by dietary ingestion or sunlight exposure. The main side effect of vitamin D toxicity is an accumulation of calcium in the blood, leading to poor appetite, nausea, vomiting, and bone pain. Sometimes, frequent urination and kidney-related problems may occur.

Extremely large doses of vitamin D need to be ingested to cause vitamin D toxicity. Supplementing with the recommended dose, or even doses that are higher than the recommended dose, is not likely to lead to vitamin D toxicity. Talk to your physician about appropriate dosing if you are planning to use larger than recommended doses of vitamin D, and she will guide you with regard to the appropriate dosage for your underlying medical conditions.

Case History (continued)

Sandy

Sandy visited her doctor to discuss omega-3 fatty acids and how they might play a role in the treatment of her condition. She was reassured that there were several benefits associated with omega-3 use, and that the form of intake did not factor heavily into the effects seen with consistent use. The main goal was to achieve a sustained target of 1 to 3 grams of EPA and DHA on a daily basis. On further questioning, Sandy admitted to enjoying fatty fish, particularly tuna and salmon; however, she could not eat these on a daily basis. Three times weekly was the typical frequency with which she ate fish. When it was suggested that Sandy supplement with around 2 grams of EPA and DHA on the days that she did not eat fish, she was agreeable to that plan. Sandy was advised to minimize omega-6 fatty acids because the inflammatory properties seen with consistent omega-6 use increased her risk for heart disease, cancer, and inflammation, which would be detrimental to a person with NAFLD.

Part 3
Healthy Liver Diet Program

12 Steps for Implementing the Program

Case History

Tara Milosovich

Tara is a 43-year-old schoolteacher. She was an avid tennis player through her teen years and well into her 20s. In fact, she had competed on the national scene for almost 10 years. She remembers what it was like to be fit and to eat nutritious meals in a controlled manner. During the past 10 years, her lifestyle has changed considerably. She has two children and is busy tending to their needs while working full time. As a consequence, Tara and her family have been eating more at restaurants, and heating up takeout or packaged meals when at home. Tara has gained almost 40 pounds (18 kg). She now has high blood pressure and nonalcoholic fatty liver disease. She knows that she needs to lose weight, and is determined to regain her previously fit form. She has researched some of the "brand name" or popular diets and feels that they are not the proper fit for her. She is not interested in rapid weight loss. Rather, maintaining a balanced nutrient intake is of importance to Tara. She does not wish to restrict any food groups, and wishes to maintain some flexibility over her eating patterns. She visited our clinic with the hope of discussing in detail possible healthy foods for her NAFLD that will ultimately assist her in weight loss ...

(continued on page 128)

Healthy Liver Diet Program Principles

- Low-calorie
- High-fiber
- Balanced food groups
- Rich in micronutrients
- Sustainable

Now that you have read about the components of a diet for managing fatty liver disease, you can bring them together to create a step-by-step, long-term diet program. There's nothing magical here — all that's needed is a determined effort to change eating habits to improve your health. Nor is there any one food that will "cure" your NAFLD. Take your time with this dietary program to ensure that it sticks. In most cases, this 12-step program will assist your body in reversing the progress of your liver condition and provide you with general good health.

12 Steps for Implementing the Program

1. Determine how many calories you require daily.
2. Set your weight loss targets.
3. Lower your calorie intake.
4. Reduce portion sizes.
5. Keep a food diary.
6. Balance the food groups.
7. Limit fruit and eliminate fruit juices and sugar-containing drinks.
8. Reduce high glycemic index grains.
9. Increase fiber intake.
10. Minimize saturated fat and maximize unsaturated fats.
11. Increase intake of chromium-rich foods and supplement with vitamin D when necessary.
12. Maintain these eating habits.
13. *Bonus:* Enjoy your food!

FAQ

Q. **What distinguishes the healthy liver diet from other diets?**

A. Have a glance back at the discussion of popular fad diets. To manage fatty liver disease, your diet should promote weight loss in a slow and steady manner, should not eliminate food groups or risk nutritional deficiencies, and should be sustainable. Most of the popular diets, however, promise almost instant weight loss — which does not last. They also often eliminate or severely restrict specific food groups that are needed for general good health, putting you at risk of developing nutrient deficiencies that can result in serious illness. In brief, they can be quick, temporary, and potentially dangerous.

The healthy liver diet is also flexible. Given that we are all unique individuals with special needs and preferences, this diet needs to be flexible so that you can develop the approach that is right for you.

Step 1: Determine How Many Calories You Require Daily

Calculating how many calories you require in your daily diet is best determined by consulting with a registered dietitian. Registered dietitians are trained to bring together the science of nutrition and the pleasures of healthy eating, so they can design sound plans to help you lose weight and stay healthy.

Determining calorie requirements can be quite challenging and feel like one of the most frustrating experiences when trying to lose weight. This would be a good time to consult with your physician or dietitian.

How to Determine Your Calorie Requirements

Determine your calorie requirements in consultation with your physician or dietitian. You can also try using several predictive equations, such as the Harris-Benedict Equation, which take into consideration age, gender, and activity level. These types of equations can overestimate your energy requirements. Your doctor and dietitian can help you with this more precisely.

Once you have determined the number of calories that you require daily to maintain your weight, you should aim to reduce that number by between 250 and 500 calories daily. It is highly likely that your current calorie intake is greater than your requirement, which would explain why your weight is higher than desirable. By using your ideal calorie requirements as a guide and by making slight adjustments to your calorie intake, you can start to make progress with regard to your weight loss.

Step 2: Set Your Weight Loss Targets

Consult with your doctor and dietitian prior to committing to this long-term dietary plan. Your doctor will help you determine your baseline risk for disease, establish current conditions that are impacted by your weight, and help you with determining your baseline anthropometric measurements — notably your BMI and waist circumference. Yes, you need to lose weight, but how much weight per week or month is realistic and safe? Remember: for every 3500 calories you remove from your diet or burn with exercise, you lose 1 pound (500 g). Weight loss of 10% of your current weight will generally lead to beneficial health outcomes.

How to Set Your Weight Loss Targets

Body mass index and waist-circumference measurements can be used to determine if you are overweight or obese, as we have seen, but these anthropometric methods can also be used to set weight loss targets. Start by checking your BMI and waist measurements again.

DID YOU KNOW?

Ideal Weight

Your ideal calorie requirement for weight maintenance and your current calorie intake are likely to be different. To initiate weight loss, try to reduce your daily calorie intake by 250 to 500 calories.

Weight loss of 10% of your current weight will generally lead to beneficial health outcomes.

BMI Target

Remember: a BMI of ≥25 is considered overweight and ≥30 is considered obese in people of Caucasian background. And don't forget that some people with NAFLD may have a normal BMI but may have abdominal obesity. (Abdominal obesity is defined by a waist circumference greater than 39.4 inches/100 cm in men, and greater than 34.6 inches/88 cm in women.) Be sure to take both measurements.

Waist Circumference Target

Compare your current waist circumference with the average healthy waist circumference for your gender. Monitor these measurements on a weekly basis as you progress with your weight loss program.

Average male healthy waist circumference: <37.6 inches (94 cm)
Average female healthy waist circumference: <32 inches (80 cm)

Week	Measurements Weight/Height	Target Body Weight	Target Waist Circumference
Week 1	Weight/Height:	BMI:	Circumference:
Week 2			
Week 3			
Week 4			
Week 5			
Week 6			
Week 7			
Week 8			

Step 3: Lower Your Calorie Intake

Lower-calorie diets are indicated for patients with fatty liver disease. To facilitate weight loss, a calorie deficit is typically necessary. In principle, the primary cause for weight gain is a positive energy balance secondary to an excess of calories, with or without low energy expenditure. The amount of weight gain is influenced by genetic, familial, and socioeconomic factors. Some factors, such as genetic predisposing factors, cannot be modified, but behavioral traits can be modified in conjunction with food choices and eating habits.

FAQ

Q. If restricting calorie intake to 2000 calories promotes weight loss, why not cut back to 1000 calories or more daily?

A. There are a number of opinions regarding what constitutes a low-calorie diet. The average person eats more than 2000 calories daily, so a diet that is less than 2000 calories daily can be considered a low-calorie diet. Very-low-calorie diets also exist. This type of diet prescribes severe calorie restriction, to less than 1000 or even 800 calories daily. This severe calorie restriction should never be followed, due to a risk of malnutrition and a micronutrient deficiency of vitamins or minerals. Severely restricting calories can compromise your health. Additionally, severe restriction of calories can change a normal metabolism into a slower metabolism, one that reflects a continuously starved state. This makes it even harder to lose weight. In fatty liver disease, rapid weight loss can make the liver disease worse. To reiterate, very-low-calorie diets with a calorie restriction of 1000 calories daily or less should be avoided.

Step 4: Reduce Portion Sizes

Many people struggle with portion sizes. One of the most important decisions we make with our food is choosing how much to eat.

FAQ

Q. What is the difference between serving size and portion size?

A. A serving size is a reference amount of food as defined by the USDA, Health Canada, or another scientific body. A portion size is the amount of food that you actually put on your plate or that you plan to eat in one meal. For example, a sandwich that includes two slices of bread is considered 1 portion, but it is also considered 2 servings — because one slice of bread equals 1 portion. Portion size is important for healthy eating. Even if you eat large portions of healthy foods, you will ultimately gain weight from fat.

Calculating Servings and Portions

It's very important to learn to read food labels and calculate the number of servings in your portion sizes. People today are eating larger portion sizes than in years past. This is in part due to food manufacturers who decide what makes up 1 portion of food in packaged and restaurant meals. These portions are not necessarily the same as the recommended serving size.

Portion sizes that were once thought to be too big for one sitting are now seen as normal. Muffins, drinks, and pasta entrées in restaurants have increased substantially in size over the years.

How to Control Portion Sizes

1. Calculate the number of calories you eat daily. Once you calculate this number, aim to eat 250 to 500 calories less than that value.

2. Determine food portions by knowing how much is in a serving of food. To help you learn, use measuring cups and spoons or a food scale in the beginning. Your skill in calculating portion sizes will grow with practice. Usually $\frac{1}{2}$ cup (125 mL) is an easy place to start for fruits and vegetables, and you can use the palm of your hand or a deck of cards as a guide for meat and fish options. Use your fist as a guide for a portion of grains (such as rice or potatoes), and use your thumbnail as a guide for the portion size of fat (margarine, butter, and oil).

3. Place food on your plate rather than eating it out of a container. We often eat more food if we cannot judge the size of the portion by looking at it critically. To help visualize, a plate can look like this: $\frac{1}{4}$ protein, $\frac{1}{4}$ grain, and $\frac{1}{2}$ vegetable.

4. Use smaller plates when serving food. Many studies have shown that people tend to eat more food if it is placed on a larger plate.

5. Learn to read food labels and adjust the nutrition information on the food label to reflect the portion size that you are consuming.

Canada's Food Guide Serving Sizes Compared to Commonly Eaten Portion Sizes

Food Item & Group	Recommended Serving Size	Common Portions
Breads and Grains		
Bread	1 slice (35 g)	2 slices (70 g)
Cereal, cold	approx $\frac{3}{4}$ cup (175 mL)	approx $1\frac{1}{2}$–2 cups (375–500 mL)
Rice, cooked	$\frac{1}{2}$ cup (125 mL)	2–3 cups (500–750 mL)
Pasta, cooked	$\frac{1}{2}$ cup (125 mL)	2–4 cups (500–1000 mL)
Bagel	$\frac{1}{2}$ small bagel (45 g)	1 large bagel (180 g)

Food Item & Group	Recommended Serving Size	Common Portions
Meat & Alternatives		
Beef steak, cooked	2½ oz (75 g)	5–8 oz (150–250 g)
Ground meat, cooked	2½ oz (75 g)	5–8 oz (150–250 g)
Eggs	2	2
Peanut butter	2 tbsp (30 mL)	2–4 tbsp (30–60 mL)
Soy tofu	¾ cup (175 mL)	1 cup (250 mL)
Milk & Dairy		
Milk	1 cup (250 mL)	1 cup (250 mL)
Cheese	1½ oz (45 g)	3–5 oz (90–150 g)

Step 5: Keep a Food Diary

Increase your awareness of your current food intake and portion sizes by tracking the foods you eat. Use the 24-hour food diary table provided to record your food choices and their correspondence to the severity of your symptoms. Keep the diary for at least 1 week, ideally for the first 4 weeks of the program.

How to Use a Diet Diary

- Record everything you consume. Look for connections between your food, your environment, and your symptoms.
- Jot down your food choices just after you eat. Don't try to recall what you ate 3 days ago. Food recall is always suspect.
- Choose a typical week to keep your food diary, so that it represents what you eat on a regular basis.
- Keep the diary for weekdays and weekend days. Your symptoms might be better or sometimes worse on a weekend. Diets can change on the weekend, as does the level of stress you may experience.
- Note portion sizes. Even if you are restricting your consumption, you still need to pay attention to your portion sizes, eating until you are about 60% to 70% full.
- Show your diary to your health-care team for their interpretation. This will enable a quicker diagnosis and lay the foundation for effective meal plans.

1-Day (or 24-Hour) Diet Diary Form

Meal/Time	What did I eat?	How much?	Notes
Breakfast			
Morning snack			
Lunch			
Afternoon snack			
Dinner			
Evening snack			

Step 6: Balance the Food Groups

There are many tools available to assist with categorizing and balancing food groups. The United States Department of Agriculture ChooseMyPlate food guide and Health Canada's Eating Well with Canada's Food Guide are excellent resources to help you determine what foods can be found in each food group and how much food you need from each food group to maintain good health. Most food guides group food items to ensure you eat a nutrient-balanced diet for general good health. Beyond the general good health offered by these food groups, they can be used therapeutically to manage various disease conditions, including fatty liver disease.

Step 7: Limit Fruit and Eliminate Fruit Juices and Sugar-Containing Drinks

Most adults should aim to eat at least 7 to 8 servings of vegetables and fruits daily. Fruits and vegetables are excellent sources of fiber and many of the micronutrients that are critical for all aspects of health. Although juices fall into this category, if you have NAFLD, you should avoid juices and instead consume the whole fruit or vegetable. Juices are highly concentrated but don't contain the other beneficial nutrient properties. A piece of fruit has fiber to help with fullness. Often the portion size of fruit in relation to juice is less, which translates into eating fewer calories.

Although fruits have many nutritive components, the sugars found in fruits can be detrimental to the liver. You will need to balance the beneficial nutrients from fruit against the detrimental effects of sugar. Try limiting your fruit choices to 2 to 3 servings daily, with the remaining servings from this group coming from vegetables.

Calories come from liquids as well as solid food. By eliminating all sugar-containing beverages, you can reduce your calorie intake substantially. Minimize your consumption of fruit juices (even natural unsweetened fruit juices), soda pops, higher-fat milks (try to use only skim or 1% milk fat), iced teas, lattes, cappuccinos, and other sweetened coffees. Avoid milkshakes and hot chocolate. In short, try to make water your beverage of choice. Regular coffees and teas with minimal milk or cream and sugar (including honey) are generally lower in calories and are more acceptable in moderation, without adversely impacting the weight loss process.

USDA Food Guide

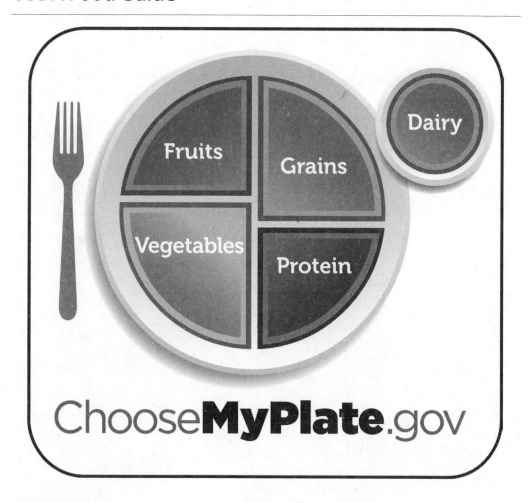

10 tips to a great plate

The USDA offer 10 tips for eating well for good health:

1. Balance calories.
2. Enjoy your food but eat less.
3. Avoid oversized portions.
4. Eat more vegetables, fruits, whole grains, and 1% dairy products (for the fatty liver diet, cap your fruit intake at 2 servings a day).
5. Make half your plate fruits and vegetables.
6. Switch to fat-free or low-fat milk.
7. Make half your grains whole grains.
8. Cut back on foods high in solid fats, added sugars, and salt.
9. Compare sodium in foods and select low-sodium or no-salt-added products.
10. Drink water instead of sugary drinks.

Eating Well with Canada's Food Guide

Recommended Number of *Food Guide Servings* per Day

	Children			Teens		Adults			
Age in Years	2-3	4-8	9-13	14-18		19-50		51+	
Sex	Girls and Boys			Females	Males	Females	Males	Females	Males
Vegetables and Fruit	4	5	6	7	8	7-8	8-10	7	7
Grain Products	3	4	6	6	7	6-7	8	6	7
Milk and Alternatives	2	2	3-4	3-4	3-4	2	2	3	3
Meat and Alternatives	1	1	1-2	2	3	2	3	2	3

What is One Food Guide Serving?
Look at the examples below.

Fresh, frozen or canned vegetables
125 mL (½ cup)

Bread
1 slice (35 g)

Bagel
½ bagel (45 g)

Milk or powdered milk (reconstituted)
250 mL (1 cup)

Cooked fish, shellfish, poultry, lean meat
75 g (2 ½ oz.)/125 mL (½ cup)

The chart above shows how many Food Guide Servings you need from each of the four food groups every day.

Having the amount and type of food recommended and following the tips in *Canada's Food Guide* will help:

- Meet your needs for vitamins, minerals and other nutrients.
- Reduce your risk of obesity, type 2 diabetes, heart disease, certain types of cancer and osteoporosis.
- Contribute to your overall health and vitality.

For the full guide, please contact Health Canada or visit their website (www.hc-sc.gc.ca).

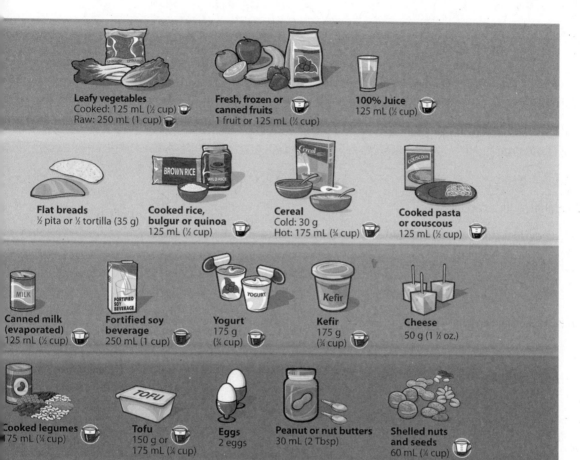

Leafy vegetables
Cooked: 125 mL (½ cup)
Raw: 250 mL (1 cup)

Fresh, frozen or canned fruits
1 fruit or 125 mL (½ cup)

100% Juice
125 mL (½ cup)

Flat breads
½ pita or ½ tortilla (35 g)

Cooked rice, bulgur or quinoa
125 mL (½ cup)

Cereal
Cold: 30 g
Hot: 175 mL (¾ cup)

Cooked pasta or couscous
125 mL (½ cup)

Canned milk (evaporated)
125 mL (½ cup)

Fortified soy beverage
250 mL (1 cup)

Yogurt
175 g
(¾ cup)

Kefir
175 g
(¾ cup)

Cheese
50 g (1 ½ oz.)

Cooked legumes
175 mL (¾ cup)

Tofu
150 g or
175 mL (¾ cup)

Eggs
2 eggs

Peanut or nut butters
30 mL (2 Tbsp)

Shelled nuts and seeds
60 mL (¼ cup)

Oils and Fats

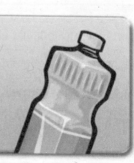

- Include a small amount – 30 to 45 mL (2 to 3 Tbsp) – of unsaturated fat each day. This includes oil used for cooking, salad dressings, margarine and mayonnaise.
- Use vegetable oils such as canola, olive and soybean.
- Choose soft margarines that are low in saturated and trans fats.
- Limit butter, hard margarine, lard and shortening.

Calories in Popular Beverages

Beverage	Serving Size	Calories
Apple juice, unsweetened	12 oz (375 mL)	169–175
Beer	12 oz (375 mL)	153
Coffee with half-and-half (10%) cream (2 tbsp/30 mL)	12 oz (375 mL)	39–43
Coffee with heavy or whipping (35%) cream (2 tbsp/30 mL)	12 oz (375 mL)	104–108
Coffee with whipped cream from can (2 tbsp/30 mL)	12 oz (375 mL)	15–19
Coffee, black	12 oz (375 mL)	0–4
Cranberry juice cocktail	12 oz (375 mL)	205
Energy drink (for example, Red Bull)	12 oz (375 mL)	160
Hard liquor (vodka, rum, whiskey, gin; 80 proof)	1½ oz (45 mL)	96
Latte, nonfat (Starbucks)	12 oz (375 mL)	120
Latte, whole milk (Starbucks)	12 oz (375 mL)	200
Milk, 1% low-fat	12 oz (375 mL)	154
Milk, 2% low-fat	12 oz (375 mL)	183
Milk, nonfat	12 oz (375 mL)	125
Milk, whole	12 oz (375 mL)	220
Orange juice, unsweetened	12 oz (375 mL)	157–168
Soda	12 oz (375 mL)	124–189
Sports drink (for example, Gatorade)	12 oz (375 mL)	94
Tea, bottled, sweet	12 oz (375 mL)	129–143
Tea, brewed, unsweetened	12 oz (375 mL)	4
Tomato/vegetable juice	12 oz (375 mL)	80
Wine, red	5 oz (150 mL)	125
Wine, white	5 oz (150 mL)	122

Step 8: Reduce High Glycemic Index Grains

Bread, bagels, rice, quinoa, cereal, pasta, and couscous are examples of grain products. Adults who are not overweight or obese and don't have NAFLD generally require 6 to 7 servings of grain products daily. Grain products are among the leading sources of carbohydrates and are required for optimal energy. However, many people tend to overeat these products, which leads to weight gain. If you have NAFLD, one method to cut down on your daily calories is to reduce your grain intake by 1 to 2 servings daily. By reducing your grain intake even by this small amount, you will be able to lose weight appropriately, without sacrificing your nutrient intake.

Step 9: Increase Fiber Intake

Higher-fiber whole-grain foods have many beneficial effects on your health and will keep you satiated, or satisfied, for a longer period of time compared to the processed and refined grains used in white breads. The bulk in fiber can help prevent overconsumption of other types of food.

Prebiotics are carbohydrate fibers that stimulate the growth of beneficial bacteria in the gut and lower the acidity in the gastrointestinal tract, which impedes the growth of bacteria that are known to predispose toward obesity and fatty liver disease. The ability of some prebiotic-containing foods, such as Jerusalem artichokes and chicory, to modulate and regulate gut bacteria has been well established.

Step 10: Minimize Saturated Fats and Maximize Unsaturated Fats

Milk and alternatives and meat and alternatives are high in saturated fats. Aim to minimize your intake of the saturated fats found in these two food groups. For example, choose lower-percentage milk fat options and limit cheese intake. Foods in the meat and alternatives category include animal-based products, such as fish, poultry, and red meats. Vegetarian sources in this category include legumes, tofu, eggs, and nuts.

Although milk and meat products are rich in protein and provide important micronutrients, they are high in saturated "bad" fats. With NAFLD, you can minimize your saturated fat intake by choosing lean cuts of meat, trimming visible fat, and using low-fat cooking methods. Maximize your intake of the unsaturated fats found in nuts, seeds, and fish, being mindful of portion sizes and servings. Unsaturated fats include omega-3 essential fatty acids, which are known to help the course of your fatty liver. Increase your intake of omega-3 EFAs to balance your intake of omega-6 fats.

Step 11: Increase Chromium-Rich Foods and Supplement with Vitamin D When Necessary

Both chromium and vitamin D have a positive effect on fatty liver disease, but adequate doses of these micronutrients are hard to obtain from natural food and sunlight sources. To assist your liver in healing, supplement with chromium and vitamin D. Consult with your doctor to determine an effective yet safe dosage.

Step 12: Maintain These Eating Habits

The greatest incentive for complying with the healthy liver diet is how great you begin to feel every day and how good your blood tests look, with little or no fat deposits in your liver. Compliance is still a challenge. The Canadian Medical Association has created a set of guidelines to help you maintain your healthy liver diet.

Canadian Medical Association Strategies for Maintaining Long-Term Weight Loss

1. *Engage in a high level of physical activity:* Women who have lost more than 70 pounds (32 kg) on average and kept it off for at least 6 years expended 2545 calories weekly in physical activity. Men expended 3293 calories weekly, which amounts to about 1 hour daily.
2. *Eat a diet that is low in calories and fat:* People with successful weight loss and who maintain that weight loss consume low-fat and low-calorie diets, with 24% of daily calories coming from fat.
3. *Eat breakfast.*
4. *Self-monitor weight on a regular basis:* Weigh yourself once weekly, using the same scale at the same time of day and wearing the same amount of clothing.
5. *Follow a consistent eating routine:* People who report a consistent diet across the week, without transgressions on the weekend, are 1.5 times more likely to maintain their weight within 5 pounds (2.5 kg) by the subsequent year — compared to people who dieted more strictly on weekdays.
6. *Catch "slips" before they turn into larger regains.*

Step 13: *Bonus:* Enjoy Your Food!

Food is a simple pleasure of life. There is no need to strip pleasure from your diet. To start, try eating healthy 80% of the time and allow a predetermined, pre-portioned treat 20% of the time. This means that on 1.5 days weekly, you can have a treat that exceeds the minimum calorie requirement. It should be planned, to avoid overeating or indulging.

FAQ

Q. Can I drink alcohol while following this healthy liver diet?

A. There are two issues to bear in mind on the issue of alcohol in the context of fatty liver disease. Alcohol consumption can lead to fatty liver disease. In fact, until the rise in obesity rates in the past 20 years or so, the overconsumption of alcohol was thought to be the most common cause of fatty liver. Drinking alcohol while you have NAFLD is generally not a good idea because it can make your liver disease worse. If you have NASH (fat plus inflammation and scarring), alcohol abstinence is mandatory. Once scarring of the liver has occurred, any liver insult that could contribute toward progression of the liver disease must be avoided.

In milder cases of NAFLD, where fat is deposited on the liver, but there is an absence of inflammation and scarring (this can only be determined from a liver biopsy result), alcohol intake is not completely contraindicated, but it must be used judiciously. This is because alcohol is one of the beverages that has minimal nutritive value but has extra calories, which can contribute to weight gain. It is best to refrain from drinking more than three standard alcoholic beverages weekly if you have mild NAFLD.

How you eat and what you eat

1. Plan your meals and snacks ahead of time. Use your meal plan to prepare your grocery list.
2. Eat slowly and chew your food thoroughly. Enjoy every mouthful. It takes your brain 15 to 20 minutes to recognize satiety, the sense that you feel full. If you rush your meal, you will tend to overeat.
3. Drink plenty of water. Your body needs fluids, and water contains no calories. You can add some flavor to water by adding a slice of fresh lemon or lime; chopped frozen fruit, such as strawberries or cranberries; vegetables, such as cucumber; ginger; herbs, such as mint or basil; or edible flowers, such as lavender or rose water.
4. Choose lower-calorie recipes. Many of your favorite foods can be prepared with fewer calories by cutting back on the fats and sugars.

5. Minimize sugar-containing beverages. These include fruit juices, soda pop, iced tea, hot chocolate, and fancy coffees, such as lattes and frappuccinos. If you must, drink low to moderate amounts of diet drinks, but be cautious about the use of artificial sweeteners. Some studies have even suggested that artificial sweeteners may have negative effects on diabetes and weight gain, but these effects are still debatable.

6. Control portion sizes and learn to understand the number of servings in a batch of food.

Case History (continued)

Tara

Tara had a discussion with her doctor concerning nutrition in NAFLD. We estimated her calorie requirement to be 1600 calories daily. She maintained a food diary for 3 days, which indicated that she was eating closer to 2100 calories daily. At this rate, she was set to gain close to 1 pound (500 g) weekly! We discussed a target of 1500 calories daily to facilitate her weight loss. It was suggested that she choose only whole-grain carbohydrate options, and to consume 4 servings of grains daily. Tara did not enjoy red meats much, and preferred fish. She was educated about the good fats in fish and how they were important to help her with heart health as well as NAFLD. She asked about healthy alternatives to fish, because her husband did not enjoy eating fish. Tara did enjoy legumes and nuts, which also offer good sources of protein and fats. She elected to avoid all beverages except water and the occasional cup of coffee, the last of which had always given her great pleasure. Lastly, she was committed to learning how to read food labels to calculate the number of servings in a portion of food, and to learn better portion control. She felt that these small changes could be incorporated into her lifestyle. They would not deprive her of nutrient-rich foods, and they would not eliminate entire food groups. Instead, they would provide her with a slow and steady weight loss of 1 pound (500 g) weekly.

Menu Plans

What is a menu plan?

A menu plan helps you choose what to eat at each meal, to ensure you are getting enough but not too many macronutrients to maintain a healthy energy level and adequate micronutrients to enable digestion and prevent nutrient deficiencies. A menu plan can support the preventive and therapeutic function of food. There are many different meal plans, but the plans presented here are designed to enable the weight loss often needed to manage fatty liver disease and to achieve basic good nutrition. There are three plans, each with 2 weeks of meals:

- 1500 calorie plan × 2 weeks
- 2000 calorie plan × 2 weeks
- 2500 calorie plan × 2 weeks

How to use a menu plan

1. Calculate your current energy intake by reviewing your food diary with your registered dietitian or physician.
2. Now drop your current energy intake by 500 calories daily.
3. Match that number as closely as possible to the 1500, 2000 or 2500 calorie meal plan. This is the menu plan you should follow to begin your healthy liver diet program.

- There may be a discrepancy between the number calculated in Step 1 and your daily required energy. This is to be expected. It is best that you work with the number you calculated in Step 1 so that you do not drop your energy intake too quickly, risk nutrient deficiencies, and find you cannot sustain weight loss.
- Remember that determining how many calories you require per day is challenging and influenced by numerous factors, including height, weight, sex, age, body composition, and activity level.
- For weight loss to occur, a calorie deficit is necessary. If you are maintaining your weight at your current level of intake and activity level, then reducing your calories by 500 calories daily will result in weight loss of about one pound per week.
- In very general terms, sedentary females would choose the 1500 calorie plan, active females and sedentary males would choose the 2000 calorie plan, and active males would choose the 2500 calorie meal plan.

1500 Calorie Meal Plan — Week 1

	Monday	Tuesday	Wednesday	
Breakfast	1 cup (250 mL) cooked Red River cereal 1 cup (250 mL) berries 1 cup (250 mL) skim milk	1 Orange Cranberry Flax Muffin* 1 cup (250 mL) low-fat, artificially sweetened flavored yogurt 1 small banana	2 boiled eggs 2 slices whole wheat toast 1 tsp (5 mL) non-hydrogenated margarine	
AM Snack		1 medium orange	1 small banana	
Lunch	1 serving Country Lentil Soup* 2 servings Spinach Fancy*	1 serving Tuna Salad Melt* 1 serving Citrus Fennel Slaw*	1 serving Vegetarian Chili* 2-oz (56 g) whole wheat roll	
PM Snack	1 small apple 2 pieces light cheese (2- x 1- x 1-inch/5 x 2.5 x 2.5 cm pieces) 4 Ryvita crackers	2 large celery stalks 2 tbsp (30 mL) low-fat salad dressing	½ cup (125 mL) cottage cheese (1%–2% M.F.) 7 pieces multi-fiber melba toast	
Supper	1 serving Chicken in Butter Sauce* ⅓ cup (75 mL) cooked rice 2 cups (500 mL) green beans, cooked	1 serving Eggplant Lasagna* 2-oz (60 g) focaccia 1 cup (250 mL) lettuce with 1 tsp (5 mL) salad dressing	1 serving Beef Tenderloin with Blue Cheese Herb Crust* 1 medium baked potato 1 cup (250 mL) broccoli, steamed	
HS Snack	1 cup (250 mL) All-Bran Buds 1 cup (250 mL) skim milk	4 gingersnap cookies ½ cup (250 mL) soy milk (chocolate or strawberry)	1 serving Chicken, Hummus and Sautéed Veggie Wraps*	

* From our list of 110 recipes

Thursday	Friday	Saturday	Sunday
1 serving Berry Smoothie* 1 bagel (3-inch/7.5 cm diameter) 2 tbsp (30 mL) light cream cheese	¾ cup (175 mL) All-Bran cereal 1 cup (250 mL) strawberries 1 cup (250 mL) skim milk	2 servings Crepes with Smoked Salmon* 1 cup (250 mL) chopped cantaloupe 2 slices whole wheat toast	1 serving Local Veggie Scrambled Eggs* 1 whole-grain English muffin
1 cup (250 mL) low-fat, artificially sweetened flavored yogurt	1 cup (250 mL) chopped grapefruit	½ cup (125 mL) grapes	½ cup (125 mL) soy milk (chocolate or strawberry)
1 serving Thai Turkey Stir-Fry* ⅔ cup (150 mL) cooked rice	2 servings Green Pea and Tarragon Soup* 2 servings Tomato Mozzarella Salad* 2-oz (56 g) whole wheat roll	3 slices low-fat beef on a small whole wheat bun 1 serving Easy Black Beans*	1 serving Pad Thai* 1 serving Beet, Orange and Jicama Salad*
1 medium pear 14 dry-roasted almonds	1 small apple 2 servings Roasted Chickpeas*	1 Ginger Cookie*	2 medium kiwifruit
1 serving Peachy Glazed Trout* 8 asparagus spears 1 serving Vegetable Quinoa Salad*	1 serving Portobello Mushroom Burgers with Cheese Filling* Tossed greens with 2 tbsp (30 mL) low-fat salad dressing	1 serving Sweet-and-Sour Pork* ⅔ cup (150 mL) cooked rice 2 servings Ginger Carrots*	1 serving Cedar-Baked Salmon* 1 serving Herbed Green Potato Salad* 1 serving Roasted Lemon Asparagus*
2 servings Piquant White Bean and Parsley Dip* ½ whole wheat pita (6 inches/15 cm)	1 serving Rice Pudding*	1 serving Blueberry Semolina Cake*	1 small banana 2 tbsp (30 mL) natural peanut butter

1500 Calorie Meal Plan — Week 2

	Monday	Tuesday	Wednesday	
Breakfast	1 serving Big-Batch Power Porridge* 1 cup (250 mL) blueberries 1 tbsp (15 mL) ground flax seeds	1 serving Berry Smoothie* 14 dry-roasted almonds	2 pieces of whole wheat toast with 2 tbsp (30 mL) natural peanut butter 1 cup (250 mL) skim milk	
AM Snack	1 cup (250 mL) low-fat, artificially sweetened flavored yogurt	1 cup (250 mL) grapes 1 serving Mango Mousse*	1 medium orange	
Lunch	¾ cup (175 mL) vegetable soup 4 servings Sardine and Pesto Spread* 7 pieces multi-fiber melba toast	1 serving Linguine with Chili Shrimp* 2 servings Greens with Strawberries*	1 serving Chickpea Curry* ⅔ cup (150 mL) cooked rice 2 servings Ginger Carrots*	
PM Snack	2 servings Bulgur and Vegetable Lettuce Wraps*			
Supper	1 serving Chicken Florentine* ⅔ cup (150 mL) cooked rice 1 cup (250 mL) Brussels sprouts, boiled	1 serving Mustard Lamb Chops* 1 serving Green Beans with Tomato Sauce* ½ cup (125 mL) mashed potatoes	1 serving Teriyaki Halibut* 1 serving Roasted Vegetables*	
HS Snack	1 small banana 2 tbsp (30 mL) natural peanut butter	1 cup (250 mL) All-Bran Buds 1 cup (250 mL) skim milk	1 serving Chicken, Hummus and Sautéed Veggie Wraps*	

* From our list of 110 recipes

Thursday	Friday	Saturday	Sunday
1 Blueberry Bran Muffin* 2 oz (60 g) light Cheddar cheese (<22% M.F.) 1 cup (250 mL) vanilla-flavored almond milk	3 shredded whole wheat biscuits 1 small banana 1 cup (250 mL) skim milk	1 serving Oatmeal Banana Pancakes* 1 tsp (5 mL) non-hydrogenated margarine 1 tbsp (15 mL) syrup 2 slices back bacon	1 serving French Toast* 1 tsp (5 mL) non-hydrogenated margarine 1 tbsp (15 mL) syrup 3 turkey sausage links (3 oz/90 g)
1 cup (250 mL) chopped grapefruit	1 cup (250 mL) chopped watermelon	1 medium orange	1 small banana
2 servings Spinach Soup* 1 serving Cornmeal Casserole*	2 servings Ham and Pineapple Pizza* 1 cup (250 mL) lettuce with 2 tsp (10 mL) olive oil and 2 tsp (10 mL) balsamic vinegar	2 servings Tasty Fish Cakes* 1 tbsp (15 mL) low-calorie tartar sauce	1 turkey and Swiss cheese sandwich 1 serving Cream of Broccoli Soup* 1 cup (250 mL) lettuce with 2 tsp (10 mL) olive oil and 2 tsp (10 mL) balsamic vinegar
		1 cup (250 mL) chopped honeydew melon	
2 servings Vegetable Moussaka*	1 serving Pork Tenderloin* 1 serving Braised Red Cabbage* 1 cup (250 mL) mashed potatoes	2 servings Beef Stew* 2-oz (60 g) focaccia	1 serving Maple Ginger Salmon* 1 serving Spinach Rice* 8 asparagus spears
½ tuna salad sandwich 1 medium tomato, sliced	1 serving Chocolate Zucchini Cake*	½ cup (125 mL) cottage cheese (1% to 2% M.F.) 1 medium tomato, sliced 7 pieces multi-fiber melba toast	1 medium apple

2000 Calorie Meal Plan — Week 1

	Monday	Tuesday	Wednesday	
Breakfast	1 cup (250 mL) whole wheat hot cereal, cooked ¼ cup (60 mL) wheat germ 1 cup (250 mL) berries 1 cup (250 mL) skim milk	1 oat bran muffin 1 cup (250 mL) plain yogurt (1% to 2% M.F.) 4 apricots	1 whole wheat English muffin with 2 oz (60 g) extra-lean ham, 1 oz (30 g) light cheese and 1 poached large egg ½ cup (125 mL) chopped mango ½ cup (250 mL) soy milk (chocolate or strawberry)	
AM Snack	2 servings Cucumber Watermelon Salad*	1 serving Berry Smoothie* 4 gingersnap cookies	1 small banana 1 tbsp (15 mL) natural peanut butter	
Lunch	1 serving Country Lentil Soup* 2-oz (56 g) whole wheat roll 1 tsp (5 mL) non-hydrogenated margarine 2 oz (60 g) light Cheddar cheese (18%)	1 serving Tuna Salad Melt* 1 serving Yam Fries* Tossed greens with 2 tbsp (30 mL) low-fat salad dressing	1 serving Tofu Patties* 1 hamburger bun 2 servings Tomato Mozzarella Salad*	
PM Snack	1 small apple 2 tbsp (30 mL) natural peanut butter 4 Ryvita crackers	3 large celery stalks ½ cup (125 mL) hummus	½ cup (125 mL) cottage cheese (1% to 2% M.F.) 7 pieces multi-fiber melba toast	
Supper	1 serving Chicken in Butter Sauce* ⅔ cup (150 mL) cooked rice 1 serving Green Beans with Tomato Sauce*	1 serving Potato-Crusted Zucchini, Carrot and Smoked Cheddar Quiche* 2-oz (60 g) focaccia 1 cup (250 mL) lettuce with 1 tsp (5 mL) salad dressing	1 serving Hamburger Soup* 1 medium baked potato 1 cup (250 mL) broccoli with 1 piece light cheese (2- x 1- x 1-inch/5 x 2.5 x 2.5 cm)	
HS Snack	1 cup (250 mL) All-Bran Buds 1 cup (250 mL) skim milk	1 Orange Cranberry Flax Muffin* 1 tsp (5 mL) non-hydrogenated margarine ½ cup (250 mL) soy milk (chocolate or strawberry)	1 serving Chicken, Hummus and Sautéed Veggie Wraps*	

* From our list of 110 recipes

Thursday	Friday	Saturday	Sunday
1 cup (250 mL) bran flakes cereal with ¼ cup (60 mL) low-fat granola 1 cup (250 mL) strawberries 1 cup (250 mL) skim milk	1 serving Berry Smoothie* 1 bagel (3-inch/7.5 cm diameter) 2 tbsp (30 mL) light cream cheese	1 serving Pumpkin Pancakes* 1 tbsp (15 mL) syrup 3 turkey sausage links (3 oz/90 g) 1 cup (250 mL) chopped honeydew melon	1 serving Local Veggie Scrambled Eggs* 1 serving Potato Latkes with Cilantro Sour Cream Topping* 1 cup (250 mL) vanilla-flavored almond milk
1 cup (250 mL) plain yogurt (1% to 2% M.F.) 1 large peach (or 1 cup/ 250 mL chopped)	1 cup (250 mL) chopped grapefruit 1 cup (250 mL) vanilla-flavored almond milk	1 cup (250 mL) grapes 1 serving Mango Mousse*	1 serving Carrot Cake* ½ cup (250 mL) soy milk (chocolate or strawberry)
1 serving Sweet-and-Sour Pork* 1 cup (250 mL) broccoli, steamed ⅔ cup (150 mL) cooked rice	2 servings Curried Coconut Chicken Soup* 2-oz (56 g) whole wheat roll 1 cup (250 mL) lettuce with 1 tsp (5 mL) salad dressing	1 serving Sunday Shepherd's Pie* 2 servings Roasted Vegetables*	1 serving Cornmeal Casserole* 1 serving Best Bean Salad*
1 medium pear 2 pieces light cheese (2- x 1- x 1-inch/5 x 2.5 x 2.5 cm pieces) 14 dry-roasted almonds	1 Blueberry Bran Muffin* 2 tbsp (30 mL) unsalted almond butter	1 Ginger Cookie*	2 servings Homemade Salsa* 12 baked tortilla chips
1 serving Teriyaki Halibut* 2 servings Roasted Lemon Asparagus* 1 serving Vegetable Quinoa Salad*	1 serving Portobello Mushroom Burgers with Cheese Filling* 2 servings Spinach and Goat Cheese Salad*	1 serving Beef Tenderloin with Blue Cheese Herb Crust* ⅔ cup (150 mL) cooked rice 2 servings Ginger Carrots*	1 serving Cedar-Baked Salmon* 1 serving Dijon Mashed Potatoes* 1 serving Roasted Vegetables*
2 servings Piquant White Bean and Parsley Dip* 1 whole wheat pita (6 inches/15 cm)	1 serving Rice Pudding* 1 cup (250 mL) raspberries	1 serving Blueberry Semolina Cake* 1 cup (250 mL) low-fat, artificially sweetened flavored yogurt	1 Applesauce Snack Cake* 1 cup (250 mL) skim milk

2000 Calorie Meal Plan — Week 2

	Monday	Tuesday	Wednesday	
Breakfast	1 serving Big-Batch Power Porridge* 1 cup (250 mL) chopped peaches 1 tbsp (15 mL) ground flax seeds 1 cup (250 mL) skim milk	2 low-fat whole wheat waffles 1 tbsp (15 mL) syrup 1 cup (250 mL) plain yogurt (1% to 2% M.F.) 1 small banana, sliced	1 whole wheat English muffin with 2 oz (60 g) low-fat turkey, 1 oz (30 g) light cheese and 1 poached large egg 1 cup (250 mL) chopped cantaloupe ½ cup (250 mL) soy milk (chocolate or strawberry)	
AM Snack	½ cup (125 mL) cottage cheese (1% to 2% M.F.) 1 cup (250 mL) blueberries	1 serving Berry Smoothie* ½ oz (14 g) pecans	1 small banana 2 tbsp (30 mL) natural peanut butter	
Lunch	1 serving Cream of Broccoli Soup* 3 servings Sardine and Pesto Spread* 14 pieces multi-fiber melba toast 1 serving Spinach and Goat Cheese Salad*	1 serving Scallop Risotto* 2-oz (60 g) focaccia 1 serving Roasted Lemon Asparagus*	1 serving Chicken, Hummus and Sautéed Veggie Wraps* 1 serving Tomato Mozzarella Salad*	
PM Snack	3 large celery stalks 2 tbsp (30 mL) unsalted almond butter	1 small apple 2 pieces light cheese (2- x 1-x 1-inch/5 x 2.5 x 2.5 cm pieces) 4 Ryvita crackers	½ cup (125 mL) cottage cheese (1%–2% M.F.) ½ cup (125 mL) unsweetened applesauce 7 pieces multi-fiber melba toast	
Supper	1½ servings Thai Turkey Stir-Fry* ⅔ cup (150 mL) cooked rice	1 serving Butternut Squash, Spinach and Feta Frittata* 1-oz (30 g) tea biscuit Tossed greens with 2 tbsp (30 mL) low-fat salad dressing 1 cup (250 mL) skim milk	1 serving Beef Stew* 1 medium baked potato 1 cup (250 mL) broccoli with 1 piece light cheese (2- x 1- x 1-inch/5 x 2.5 x 2.5 cm)	
HS Snack	1 serving Fresh Berry Trifle* 14 dry-roasted almonds	1 Orange Cranberry Flax Muffin* 1 tbsp (15 mL) unsalted almond butter	⅔ cup (150 mL) multigrain Cheerios 1 cup (250 mL) blueberries 1 cup (250 mL) skim milk	

* From our list of 110 recipes

Thursday	Friday	Saturday	Sunday
1 Blueberry Bran Muffin* 4 tsp (20 mL) unsalted almond butter 1 cup (250 mL) strawberries 1 cup (250 mL) skim milk	1 serving Berry Smoothie* 1 bagel (3-inch/7.5 cm diameter) 2 tbsp (30 mL) light cream cheese	1 serving Local Veggie Scrambled Eggs* 2 slices back bacon 1 slice whole wheat toast 1 tsp (5 mL) non-hydrogenated margarine 1 cup (250 mL) chopped honeydew melon	1 serving French Toast* 1 tsp (5 mL) non-hydrogenated margarine 1 tbsp (15 mL) syrup 3 turkey sausage links (3 oz/90 g) 1 cup (250 mL) chopped grapefruit 1 cup (250 mL) vanilla-flavored almond milk
1 serving Rice Pudding* 1 cup (250 mL) blackberries	1 cup (250 mL) grapes 1 cup (250 mL) vanilla-flavored almond milk	2 medium kiwifruit 1 serving Mango Mousse*	1 serving Carrot Cake* $1/2$ cup (250 mL) soy milk (chocolate or strawberry)
2 servings Country Lentil Soup* 1 serving Cornmeal Casserole* 2 servings Greens with Strawberries*	1 serving Mustard Lamb Chops* 1 serving Spaghetti Squash with Mushrooms*	1 serving Tasty Fish Cakes* 1 tbsp (15 mL) low-calorie tartar sauce 1 serving Herbed Green Potato Salad* 1 serving Spinach and Goat Cheese Salad*	2 servings Ham and Pineapple Pizza* 2 servings Greens with Strawberries*
1 medium pear 2 pieces light cheese (2- x 1- x 1-inch/5 x 2.5 x 2.5 cm pieces) 14 dry-roasted almonds	1 slice rye toast 2 tbsp (30 mL) unsalted almond butter 1 cup (250 mL) skim milk	2 low-fat whole wheat waffles 1 tbsp (15 mL) syrup 1 cup (250 mL) raspberries	2 servings Homemade Salsa* 12 baked tortilla chips
1 serving Peachy Glazed Trout* $1/3$ cup (75 mL) cooked rice 1 serving Vegetable Quinoa Salad*	1 serving Portobello Mushroom Burgers with Cheese Filling* 1 serving Yam Fries* Tossed greens with 2 tbsp (30 mL) low-fat salad dressing	1 serving Beef Tenderloin with Blue Cheese Herb Crust* $2/3$ cup (150 mL) cooked rice 2 servings Ginger Carrots*	1 serving Oven-Baked Fish and Chips* 1 cup (250 mL) broccoli with 1 piece light cheese (2- x 1- x 1-inch/5 x 2.5 x 2.5 cm)
2 servings Piquant White Bean and Parsley Dip* 1 whole wheat pita (6 inches/15 cm)	3 servings Bulgur and Vegetable Lettuce Wraps*	1 serving Chocolate Zucchini Cake* 1 cup (250 mL) low-fat, artificially sweetened flavored yogurt	1 Applesauce Snack Cake* 1 cup (250 mL) skim milk

2500 Calorie Meal Plan — Week 1

	Monday	Tuesday	Wednesday	
Breakfast	1½ cups (375 mL) All-Bran cereal 1 cup (250 mL) strawberries 1½ cups (375 mL) skim milk	2 servings Berry Smoothie* 2 slices whole wheat toast 2 tsp (10 mL) non-hydrogenated margarine	3 boiled eggs 1 bagel (4½-inch/11 cm diameter) 2 tsp (10 mL) non-hydrogenated margarine	
AM Snack	1 medium orange	1 cup (250 mL) low-fat, artificially sweetened flavored yogurt		
Lunch	2 servings Egg Lemon Soup* 5 oz (150 g) skinless chicken breast, roasted 1 cup (250 mL) Brussels sprouts, boiled	2 servings Stir-Fried Scallops with Curried Sweet Peppers* ⅔ cup (150 mL) cooked rice	2 servings Vegetable Moussaka* 2 servings Tomato Mozzarella Salad*	
PM Snack	1 cup (250 mL) cottage cheese (1% to 2% M.F.) 14 pieces multi-fiber melba toast	1 serving Chicken, Hummus and Sautéed Veggie Wraps*	1½ cups (375 mL) All-Bran Buds 1½ cups (375 mL) skim milk	
Supper	2 servings Spicy Brown Rice Jambalaya* 2-oz (56 g) whole wheat roll	1 serving Pork Tenderloin* 1 serving Dijon Mashed Potatoes* 2 servings Quick and Delicious Maple Squash*	1 serving Brined and Tender Lemon Roast Chicken* 1 medium potato, roasted 2 servings Green Beans with Tomato Sauce*	
HS Snack	1 large banana 3 tbsp (45 mL) natural peanut butter	6 gingersnap cookies 4 medium kiwifruit		

* From our list of 110 recipes

Thursday	Friday	Saturday	Sunday
1½ cups (375 mL) cooked Red River cereal 2 cups (500 mL) berries 2 cups (500 mL) skim milk	2 Orange Cranberry Flax Muffins* 1 cup (250 mL) low-fat, artificially sweetened flavored yogurt 1 large banana	1 serving Local Veggie Scrambled Eggs* 2 slices whole wheat toast 2 tsp (10 mL) non-hydrogenated margarine	2 servings Pumpkin Pancakes* 2 tbsp (30 mL) syrup 3 turkey sausage links (3 oz/90 g)
2 servings Rice Pudding*	1 medium apple	1 cup (250 mL) chopped grapefruit	1 large banana
2 servings Mustard Lamb Chops* 1 serving Braised Red Cabbage* ½ medium potato, boiled	2 servings Curried Coconut Chicken Soup* 1 tuna salad sandwich 1 cup (250 mL) lettuce with 2 tsp (10 mL) olive oil and 2 tsp (10 mL) balsamic vinegar	1 serving Pasta with White Clam Sauce* 2 cups (500 mL) lettuce with 1 tbsp (15 mL) olive oil and 1 tbsp (15 mL) balsamic vinegar 2-oz (56 g) whole wheat roll	1 serving Tofu Patties* 1 hamburger bun 2 servings Best Bean Salad*
2 servings Piquant White Bean and Parsley Dip* 1 whole wheat pita (6 inches/15 cm)	2 servings Vegetarian Chili*	1 medium pear 14 pieces multi-fiber melba toast 2 oz (60 g) light Cheddar cheese (18%)	½ can (6 oz/170 g) canned sockeye salmon, drained, with bones 10 Triscuits
1 serving Teriyaki Halibut* ⅔ cup (150 mL) cooked rice 2 servings Cucumber Watermelon Salad*	5 oz (150 g) roasted top round beef, fat trimmed 1 serving Roasted Vegetables* 1 serving Yam Fries*	2 servings Chickpea Curry* 1 cup (250 mL) cooked couscous 2 servings Ginger Carrots*	1 serving Oven-Baked Fish and Chips* 1 cup (250 mL) peas and carrots, boiled
1 small apple 4 pieces light cheese (2- x 1- x 1-inch/5 x 2.5 x 2.5 cm pieces) 4 Ryvita crackers	4 servings Sardine and Pesto Spread* 2 slices pumpernickel bread	4 large celery stalks 2 tbsp (30 mL) unsalted almond butter	2 Blueberry Bran Muffins* 1 cup (250 mL) chopped mango

2500 Calorie Meal Plan — Week 2

	Monday	Tuesday	Wednesday	
Breakfast	1 cup (250 mL) Kashi Honey Almond Flax Flavor cereal 1 cup (250 mL) blueberries 1½ cups (375 mL) skim milk	1 serving Berry Smoothie* 1 whole wheat English muffin with 2 oz (60 g) low-fat turkey, 1 oz (30 g) light cheese and 1 poached large egg 1 medium orange	1 serving Big-Batch Power Porridge* 2 cups (500 mL) berries 2 cups (500 mL) skim milk	
AM Snack	1 cup (250 mL) cubed papaya 1 cup (250 mL) plain yogurt (1% to 2% M.F.)	1½ cups (375 mL) low-fat, artificially sweetened flavored yogurt 4 arrowroot cookies	3 servings Sardine and Pesto Spread* 10 Triscuits	
Lunch	5 oz (150 g) skinless chicken breast, roasted 1 serving Spicy Brown Rice Jambalaya* 2 cups (500 mL) lettuce with 1 tbsp (15 mL) olive oil and 1 tbsp (15 mL) balsamic vinegar	2 servings Scallop Risotto* 2 servings Green Beans with Tomato Sauce*	2 servings Tofu Patties* 1 hamburger bun 2 servings Tomato Mozzarella Salad*	
PM Snack	1 cup (250 mL) cottage cheese (1% to 2% M.F.) 14 pieces multi-fiber melba toast	1 Blueberry Bran Muffin* ¼ cup (60 mL) light cream cheese	3 servings Roasted Chickpeas* 1 cup (250 mL) vanilla-flavored almond milk	
Supper	2 servings Vegetarian Chili* 2-oz (56 g) whole wheat roll 1 tsp (5 mL) non-hydrogenated margarine ½ cup (250 mL) soy milk (chocolate or strawberry)	1 serving Mustard Lamb Chops* 1 serving Spaghetti Squash with Mushrooms* 1 serving Dijon Mashed Potatoes*	1 serving Chicken Florentine* ⅔ cup (150 mL) cooked rice 2 servings Roasted Lemon Asparagus* 1½ cups (375 mL) skim milk	
HS Snack	2 low-fat whole wheat waffles 1 tbsp (15 mL) syrup 2 tbsp (30 mL) natural peanut butter	1 serving Carrot Cake* 1 cup (250 mL) grapes 1½ cups (375 mL) skim milk	1 small apple 4 pieces light cheese (2- x 1- x 1-inch/5 x 2.5 x 2.5 cm pieces)	

* From our list of 110 recipes

Thursday	Friday	Saturday	Sunday
1½ cups (375 mL) All-Bran Buds 1 cup (250 mL) strawberries 2 cups (500 mL) skim milk	2 Orange Cranberry Flax Muffins* 1 cup (250 mL) plain yogurt (1% to 2% M.F.) 1 cup (250 mL) chopped peaches	1 serving Local Veggie Scrambled Eggs* 2 slices back bacon 1 bagel (3-inch/7.5 cm diameter) 2 tbsp (30 mL) light cream cheese	1 serving Oatmeal Banana Pancakes* 2 tbsp (30 mL) syrup 3 turkey sausage links (3 oz/90 g) 1 cup (250 mL) raspberries
1 serving Berry Smoothie* ¼ oz (7 g) pecans	2 servings Piquant White Bean and Parsley Dip* 1 whole wheat pita (6 inches/15 cm)	1 serving French Toast* 2 tbsp (30 mL) syrup 1 cup (250 mL) chopped grapefruit	3 Ginger Cookies* 1 cup (250 mL) plain yogurt (1% to 2% M.F.)
1 serving Pork Tenderloin* 1 serving Braised Red Cabbage* 1 serving Herbed Green Potato Salad*	2 servings Hot and Sour Chicken Soup* 2-oz (56 g) whole wheat roll 1 tsp (5 mL) non-hydrogenated margarine ½ cup (250 mL) soy milk (chocolate or strawberry)	1 serving Eggplant Lasagna* 2-oz (60 g) focaccia 2 cups (500 mL) lettuce with 1 tbsp (15 mL) olive oil and 1 tbsp (15 mL) balsamic vinegar	1 serving Potato-Crusted Zucchini, Carrot and Smoked Cheddar Quiche* 2 servings Best Bean Salad*
2 servings Homemade Salsa* 20 baked tortilla chips	½ can (6 oz/170 g) canned sockeye salmon, drained, with bones 10 Triscuits 1 medium tomato, sliced	1 medium pear 2 pieces light cheese (2- x 1- x 1-inch/5 x 2.5 x 2.5 cm pieces) 14 dry-roasted almonds	1 serving Chicken, Hummus and Sautéed Veggie Wraps*
1 serving Oven-Baked Fish and Chips* 1 serving Citrus Fennel Slaw*	1 serving Portobello Mushroom Burgers with Cheese Filling* 1 serving Yam Fries*	1 serving Thai Turkey Stir-Fry* 1 cup (250 mL) cooked couscous	1 serving Maple Ginger Salmon* 1 serving Dijon Mashed Potatoes* 1 cup (250 mL) broccoli with 1 piece light cheese (2- x 1- x 1-inch/5 x 2.5 x 2.5 cm)
4 large celery stalks ¼ cup (60 mL) unsalted almond butter	1½ cups (375 mL) cooked Red River cereal 1 small banana 1 cup (250 mL) skim milk	1 serving Rice Pudding* 1 tbsp (15 mL) ground flax seeds 1 cup (250 mL) blackberries	1 Blueberry Bran Muffin* 1½ cups (375 mL) skim milk

Part 4

Recipes for NAFLD

Introduction to the Recipes

Healthy eating with NAFLD can be an art. Its success depends on consistent lifestyle changes involving diet and exercise. We have chosen tasty and nutritious recipes to fit within the dietary recommendations for treating NAFLD. Our recipe choices and meal plans are focused on increasing total and prebiotic fiber, monounsaturated fats, polyunsaturated fats such as omega-3 fatty acids, and vitamin D in your diet while providing the optimal calories for promoting healthy weight loss. We have selected basic recipes from the culturally diverse North American kitchen, using easy-to-find ingredients. These recipes may also be a helpful guide for adapting your own favorite recipes into NAFLD-friendly versions.

Fiber

Dietary fiber is found mainly in fruits, vegetables, whole-grain products, and legumes. In particular, prebiotic fiber reduces the liver's ability to make fat. Our recipes and meal plans include garlic, leeks, onions, asparagus, wheat bran, whole wheat flour, and bananas, which are some of the best sources of prebiotic fiber.

Healthy Fats

Polyunsaturated fats are found mainly in safflower, sunflower, corn, and soybean oils and soft margarines made from these oils. Omega-3 fatty acids are also a type of polyunsaturated fat. Monounsaturated fats are found mostly in olive and canola oils and soft margarines made from these oils.

Our recipes and meal plans emphasize the use of vegetable oils and fatty fish. We have included sardines, salmon, halibut, tuna, and cod in our recipes to increase the amount of omega-3 fatty acids in your diet.

It is important to consider both the amount of fat you eat and the type of fat you eat. Minimize saturated fats from animal food sources, such as butter, meat, and fat-containing dairy products, and trans fats, from processed food. Choose healthier monounsaturated and polyunsaturated fats when preparing or cooking foods.

Vitamin D

Certain food sources provide modest doses of vitamin D. Dietary sources of vitamin D in our recipes and meal plans include salmon, tuna, sardines, orange juice, milk, yogurt, margarine, and eggs.

Breakfasts

Bircher Muesli

A great low-fat breakfast choice that is ready to eat in the morning if prepared the night before. It can be made ahead and it stores well, refrigerated, for 2 to 3 days. Garnish with fresh seasonal fruit if desired.

⅔ cup	quick-cooking rolled oats	150 mL
2 cups	2% milk	500 mL
¼ cup	granulated sugar	60 mL
¼ tsp	ground cinnamon	1 mL
1½ cups	low-fat plain yogurt	375 mL
1½ tsp	freshly squeezed lemon juice	7 mL
2	apples (unpeeled)	2
2	bananas	2

1. In a bowl, stir oats into milk; let stand for 15 minutes. Stir in sugar and cinnamon.

2. Combine yogurt and lemon juice. Dice apples; stir into yogurt mixture. Stir into softened oats. Refrigerate.

3. At serving time, slice bananas and stir into mixture.

This recipe courtesy of chefs Blair Woodruff and Kurt Zwingli, and dietitian Cathy Thibault.

Nutrients
PER SERVING

Calories	208
Fat	3 g
Carbohydrate	39 g
Fiber	2 g
Protein	8 g

Big-Batch Power Porridge

This heart-healthy recipe is not only nutritious, but will fill you up!

Tips

Look for 9-grain cereal in the bulk food store or the bulk food section of your grocery store.

Wheat germ provides 3.5 g of fiber per ¼ cup (60 mL).

To toast wheat germ, heat a skillet over medium heat, add wheat germ and toast gently, shaking occasionally to ensure even toasting, for about 4 minutes or until fragrant.

Add brown sugar and warmed milk; also delicious with a handful of blueberries.

6 cups	large-flake old-fashioned rolled oats	1.5 L
1 cup	9-grain cereal (such as Red River)	250 mL
¾ cup	wheat germ, toasted (see tip, at left)	175 mL
½ cup	oat bran	125 mL
½ cup	raisins or dried cranberries	125 mL
½ cup	sunflower seeds	125 mL

1. In a large bowl, combine oats, 9-grain cereal, wheat germ, oat bran, raisins and sunflower seeds. Store in a large covered container at room temperature for up to 1 week or in the refrigerator for up to 3 months.

2. To prepare 1 serving, bring 1 cup (250 mL) water to a boil in a small saucepan. Add ½ cup (125 mL) porridge mixture; stir and reduce heat to low. Cook, stirring occasionally, for about 5 minutes or until thickened.

This recipe courtesy of Konnie Kranenburg.

Nutrients
PER SERVING

Calories	201
Fat	5 g
Carbohydrate	33 g
Fiber	5 g
Protein	9 g

Local Veggie Scrambled Eggs

Makes 6 servings

A Mediterranean-inspired recipe to please the taste buds and provide energy.

Tips

Canola oil contains healthy omega-3 fats.

If you're short on time, you can use store-bought tzatziki instead of homemade.

8	eggs	8
¼ cup	Homemade Tzatziki (see recipe, below)	60 mL
½ cup	crumbled feta cheese	125 mL
1 tsp	dried oregano	5 mL
½ tsp	freshly ground black pepper	2 mL
2 tsp	canola oil	10 mL
½ cup	finely chopped green onions	125 mL
½ cup	chopped cooked potato	125 mL
½ cup	chopped roasted red bell peppers	125 mL
½ cup	chopped lightly steamed asparagus	125 mL

1. In a medium bowl, whisk together eggs, tzatziki, feta, oregano and pepper; set aside.

2. In a large nonstick skillet, heat oil over medium heat. Sauté green onions and potato for 4 to 5 minutes or until lightly browned. Add roasted peppers and asparagus; sauté until heated through.

3. Pour in egg mixture and cook, stirring with a wooden spoon, for 2 to 3 minutes or until eggs form soft, thick curds.

This recipe courtesy of dietitian Mary Sue Waisman.

Homemade Tzatziki: Line a sieve with cheesecloth and set over a bowl. Pour in 2 cups (500 mL) plain yogurt (gelatin- and starch-free). Cover and refrigerate; let drain for 1 to 3 hours or until yogurt is thickened. Discard liquid in bowl. In a small bowl, combine drained yogurt, ½ cup (125 mL) drained grated cucumber and 2 cloves pressed garlic. Cover tightly with plastic wrap and refrigerate for at least 30 minutes or for up to 1 day.

Nutrients
PER SERVING

Calories	204
Fat	12 g
Carbohydrate	10 g
Fiber	1 g
Protein	12 g

Oatmeal Banana Pancakes

These tasty pancakes are easy to make. Top them with fresh fruit, then drizzle with maple syrup or top with dollops of yogurt.

Tips

Oat flakes are a good source of soluble fiber, offering 1.5 g per 1 cup (250 mL).

Remember to always eat breakfast. Eating breakfast will keep you feeling full for a longer period of time, lowering your risk of snacking on undesirable foods.

- **Large skillet, lightly sprayed with nonstick cooking spray**

1 cup	old-fashioned (large-flake) rolled oats	250 mL
1 cup	all-purpose flour	250 mL
1/4 cup	golden cane sugar	60 mL
1 1/2 tsp	baking powder	7 mL
1/2 tsp	baking soda	2 mL
1/2 tsp	ground cinnamon	2 mL
3/4 cup	plain yogurt	175 mL
3/4 cup	unsweetened almond milk or skim milk	175 mL
2	eggs	2
1 tsp	vanilla extract	5 mL
2	ripe bananas, mashed	2
1/4 cup	soft margarine, melted	60 mL

1. In a medium bowl, whisk together oats, flour, golden cane sugar, baking powder, baking soda and cinnamon until combined. Set aside.

2. In another medium bowl, whisk together yogurt, almond milk, eggs and vanilla until blended. Gradually stir oat mixture into yogurt mixture until just blended. Fold in bananas and margarine.

3. Into prepared skillet, over medium heat, pour one-eighth of the batter for each pancake. Cook, turning once when bubbles form on top, for about 2 minutes or until golden brown. Repeat with remaining batter.

Nutrients
PER SERVING

Calories	213
Fat	6 g
Carbohydrate	36 g
Fiber	4 g
Protein	4 g

Pumpkin Pancakes

*Get an extra fruit serving
while enjoying a fall
weekend classic.*

Tips

Pumpkin is a good source
of fiber.

You can cook your own
pie pumpkin to make the
purée for this recipe or you
can use canned pumpkin
purée; just be sure not to
use pumpkin pie filling,
which is sweetened.

The chemical reaction of
baking soda and vinegar
makes this pancake
batter particularly fluffy.
Work quickly.

- **Preheat oven to 200°F (100°C)**

1 cup	all-purpose flour	250 mL
1 cup	whole wheat flour	250 mL
3 tbsp	lightly packed brown sugar	45 mL
2 tsp	baking powder	10 mL
1 tsp	baking soda	5 mL
1 tsp	ground allspice	5 mL
1 tsp	ground cinnamon	5 mL
1/2 tsp	ground ginger	2 mL
1/4 tsp	salt	1 mL
1	egg	1
1 1/2 cups	1% milk	375 mL
1 cup	pumpkin purée (see tip, at left)	250 mL
2 tbsp	canola oil	30 mL
1 tbsp	white vinegar	15 mL
	Vegetable cooking spray	

1. In a large bowl, combine all-purpose flour, whole wheat flour, brown sugar, baking powder, baking soda, allspice, cinnamon, ginger and salt.

2. In another large bowl, whisk together egg, milk, pumpkin purée, oil and vinegar. Add to flour mixture and stir to combine.

3. Heat a griddle or large nonstick skillet over medium heat. Spray lightly with cooking spray. For each pancake, pour 1/4 cup (60 mL) batter onto griddle and cook for about 2 minutes or until bubbly around the edges. Flip and cook for 2 minutes or until golden brown. Transfer to a plate and keep warm in preheated oven. Repeat with the remaining batter, spraying griddle and adjusting heat between batches as needed.

This recipe courtesy of dietitian Karen Omichinski.

Nutrients
PER 2 PANCAKES

Calories	179
Fat	5 g
Carbohydrate	30 g
Fiber	3 g
Protein	6 g

Potato Latkes with Cilantro Sour Cream Topping

Makes 8 servings

This is a creative and delicious twist on a traditional potato treat.

Tip

Potatoes are a source of soluble fiber.

- **Food processor, fitted with grating wheel (optional)**

Cilantro Sour Cream Topping

1 cup	low-fat sour cream	250 mL
1½ tbsp	chopped fresh cilantro	22 mL
1½ tbsp	freshly squeezed lime juice	22 mL
½ tsp	salt	2 mL
½ tsp	freshly ground black pepper	2 mL

Potato Latkes

2 lbs	russet potatoes, peeled	1 kg
2	eggs	2
1 tbsp	canola or olive oil	15 mL
1 tsp	freshly squeezed lemon juice	5 mL
3 tbsp	potato flour	45 mL
1 tsp	salt	5 mL
¼ tsp	freshly ground black pepper	1 mL
	Vegetable oil, for frying	

1. *Cilantro Sour Cream Topping:* In a small bowl, stir together sour cream, cilantro, lime juice, salt and pepper. Cover and refrigerate until ready to serve.

2. *Potato Latkes:* Using food processor or a box grater, grate potatoes. Set aside.

3. In a large bowl, beat eggs. Stir in potatoes, oil and lemon juice. Stir in potato flour, salt and pepper until potatoes are uniformly coated.

4. In a large griddle or skillet, heat 1 to 2 tbsp (15 to 30 mL) oil over high heat. Spoon about 1 tbsp (15 mL) of the potato mixture into the griddle for each latke, then flatten with the back of the spoon. Cook, turning once halfway through, for 3 to 4 minutes per side or until golden brown and crisp. Transfer to paper towels and let drain. Repeat with remaining potato mixture.

5. Arrange latkes on a platter or individual serving plates and top with cilantro sour cream topping. Serve immediately.

Nutrients
PER SERVING

Calories	197
Fat	8 g
Carbohydrate	26 g
Fiber	2 g
Protein	5 g

Crêpes with Smoked Salmon

*This crêpe recipe is
simple and works
perfectly every time.*

Tips

To avoid overcooking
crêpes, cook them only
until they lose their raw
appearance, when the
batter turns from wet-
looking to dry-looking.

These crêpes can be
made ahead and frozen.
If you place waxed paper
between them before
freezing, it's easier to thaw
them one at a time. To thaw,
transfer to the refrigerator
1 to 2 hours before use.

Variation

Add a sprig of fresh dill
and a sprinkle of lemon
juice on top of the salmon
before folding.

- **6-inch (15 cm) crêpe pan or nonstick skillet**

Crêpes

2	eggs	2
1¼ cups	1% milk	300 mL
Pinch	salt	Pinch
1 cup	all-purpose flour	250 mL
	Vegetable cooking spray	

Filling

3 tbsp	herb-and-garlic-flavored cream cheese, divided	45 mL
1 cup	packed baby spinach leaves	250 mL
8 to 10	thin slices smoked salmon	8 to 10

1. *Crêpes:* In a small bowl, whisk together eggs, milk and salt. Whisk in flour until batter is blended and smooth. Cover and let rest at room temperature for 30 minutes.

2. Heat crêpe pan over medium heat. Spray lightly with cooking spray. Lift the pan and pour in about ¼ cup (60 mL) batter. Swirl the pan so the batter reaches the edges. Return to heat and cook for about 30 seconds or until crêpe is no longer shiny on top and is very light golden on the bottom. Flip and cook for 20 to 30 seconds or until starting to turn golden. Transfer to a plate, cover with foil and keep warm. Repeat with the remaining batter, spraying pan and adjusting heat between batches as needed.

3. *Filling:* Spread 1 tsp (5 mL) cream cheese over each crêpe. Place a few spinach leaves in the middle, followed by 1 slice smoked salmon. Fold bottom edge of crêpe over salmon, then fold top edge over bottom edge. Transfer to a serving plate, seam side down.

This recipe courtesy of Martine Laroche, Alberta.

Nutrients PER CRÊPE	
Calories	131
Fat	5 g
Carbohydrate	12 g
Fiber	1 g
Protein	9 g

French Toast

This classic, quick breakfast never disappoints.

Tip

Choose lower-fat milk, such as skim milk, 1% or 2%. The nutrient analysis for this recipe is based on 2% milk.

2	eggs	2
⅔ cup	2% milk	150 mL
2 tsp	vanilla extract	10 mL
½ tsp	ground cinnamon	2 mL
½ tsp	ground nutmeg	2 mL
	Salt	
6	slices Italian or French bread	6
1 tsp	soft margarine	5 mL
	Pure maple syrup, yogurt or fresh fruit	

1. In a small bowl, whisk together eggs, milk, vanilla, cinnamon, nutmeg and salt to taste. Transfer to a wide shallow dish and set aside.

2. In griddle, over medium-high heat, melt margarine.

3. Using a fork, pierce each slice of bread all over. Working in batches, dunk each slice into egg mixture for just a few seconds, turning to coat, and transfer to griddle. Cook, turning once, for about 2 minutes per side or until golden brown. Serve immediately, with your choice of toppings.

Nutrients
PER SERVING

Calories	141
Fat	6 g
Carbohydrate	13 g
Fiber	1 g
Protein	6 g

Blueberry Bran Muffins

These fiber-rich muffins are made with wheat bran, which will fill you up and can help you lose weight.

Tips

Wheat bran is an excellent source of fiber, providing 11.4 g per ¼ cup (60 mL).

These muffins freeze well. Wrap cooled muffins individually in plastic wrap, then seal in an airtight container or freezer bag and freeze for up to 1 month.

Variation

Use your favorite fruit, such as raspberries or chopped peaches, in place of the blueberries.

- **Preheat oven to 400°F (200°C)**
- **12-cup muffin pan, lightly greased or lined with paper cups**

1½ cups	wheat bran	375 mL
½ cup	all-purpose flour	125 mL
½ cup	wheat germ	125 mL
1 tsp	baking powder	5 mL
½ tsp	baking soda	2 mL
½ cup	lightly packed brown sugar	125 mL
2	eggs, beaten	2
1 cup	1% milk	250 mL
¼ cup	canola oil	60 mL
¼ cup	light (fancy) molasses	60 mL
1 cup	fresh or frozen blueberries	250 mL

1. In a large bowl, combine bran, flour, wheat germ, baking powder and baking soda.

2. In a medium bowl, whisk together brown sugar, eggs, milk, oil and molasses until blended. Pour over flour mixture and stir until just combined. Fold in blueberries.

3. Divide batter evenly among prepared muffin cups. Bake in preheated oven for 15 to 17 minutes or until tops are firm to the touch and a tester inserted in the center of a muffin comes out clean. Let cool in pan on a wire rack for 10 minutes, then transfer to rack to cool completely.

This recipe courtesy of Nancy Morgan.

Nutrients
PER MUFFIN

Calories	175
Fat	6 g
Carbohydrate	28 g
Fiber	4 g
Protein	5 g

Orange Cranberry Flax Muffins

Be kind to your heart and waistline. Enjoy a flax-filled muffin rich in fiber and omega-3s.

Tips

Ground flax seeds are a source of omega-3 fatty acids.

Assemble the wet and dry ingredients in separate bowls the night before, so it takes less than a minute to finish the prep work in the morning. Be sure to refrigerate the wet ingredients.

These muffins freeze well. Wrap cooled muffins individually in plastic wrap, then seal in an airtight container or freezer bag and freeze for up to 1 month.

Variation

Substitute dried cherries or dried blueberries for the cranberries.

- Preheat oven to 375°F (190°C)
- Two 12-cup muffin pans, 18 cups lightly greased or lined with paper cups

¾ cup	dried cranberries, coarsely chopped	175 mL
1½ cups	orange juice, divided	375 mL
2 cups	all-purpose flour	500 mL
¾ cup	whole wheat flour	175 mL
½ cup	ground flax seeds (flaxseed meal)	125 mL
½ cup	granulated sugar	125 mL
2 tsp	grated orange zest	10 mL
2 tsp	baking powder	10 mL
1 tsp	baking soda	5 mL
1	egg, beaten	1
¼ cup	canola oil	60 mL

1. In a small bowl, combine cranberries and ¼ cup (60 mL) of the orange juice. Set aside.

2. In a large bowl, combine all-purpose flour, whole wheat flour, flax seeds, sugar, orange zest, baking powder and baking soda.

3. In a medium bowl, whisk together egg, oil and the remaining orange juice until blended. Pour over flour mixture and stir until just combined. Fold in cranberry mixture.

4. Divide batter evenly among prepared muffin cups. Bake in preheated oven for 16 to 18 minutes or until tops are firm to the touch and a tester inserted in the center of a muffin comes out clean. Let cool in pans on a wire rack for 10 minutes, then transfer to rack to cool completely.

This recipe courtesy of dietitian Joan Rew.

Nutrients
PER MUFFIN

Calories	162
Fat	5 g
Carbohydrate	27 g
Fiber	2 g
Protein	3 g

Berry Smoothie

Makes 3½ to 4 cups (875 mL to 1 L)

Frozen fruits add intense flavor to a smoothie and keep it cold longer.

Tips

Yogurts labeled 2% M.F. or lower are considered low-fat options.

Freeze leftover smoothies in ice pop containers for a quick frozen treat.

Pour the smoothie into attractive wineglasses and garnish each with a fresh strawberry to serve at a weekend brunch.

Variation

Vary the frozen fruits, yogurt and juice to suit your taste. For example, try a combination of frozen mangos, frozen peaches, peach-flavored yogurt and orange juice.

• **Blender**

1	banana, broken into chunks	1
2 cups	mixed frozen berries (strawberries, blueberries, blackberries, raspberries)	500 mL
1 cup	low-fat strawberry-flavored yogurt	250 mL
1 cup	unsweetened orange, strawberry and banana juice	250 mL

1. In blender, on high speed, blend banana, berries, yogurt and juice for 30 seconds or until smooth.

This recipe courtesy of dietitian Joëlle Zorzetto.

Nutrients	
PER 1 CUP (250 ML)	
Calories	153
Fat	1 g
Carbohydrate	33 g
Fiber	3 g
Protein	4 g

Snacks, Sandwiches and Pizza

Roasted Chickpeas

*Roasted chickpeas make
a nice savory snack
alternative to chips.*

Tips

Chickpeas are low in fat
and a great source of
dietary fiber.

Be sure to drain and rinse
the chickpeas to remove
excess sodium. Pat them
dry so the coating adheres.

These can be stored in an
airtight container at room
temperature for 1 week,
but they likely won't last
that long!

Variation

Vary the spices to your
liking; added cayenne
pepper will give them a
hot kick.

- Preheat oven to 350°F (180°C)
- Baking sheet, lined with foil

1	can (19 oz/540 mL) chickpeas, rinsed, drained and patted dry	1
1 tbsp	canola oil	15 mL
½ tsp	chili powder	2 mL
¼ tsp	garlic powder	1 mL
¼ tsp	ground cumin	1 mL

1. In a small bowl, combine chickpeas, oil, chili powder, garlic powder and cumin. Stir to coat well. Spread evenly on preparing baking sheet.

2. Bake in preheated oven, stirring occasionally, for 60 to 75 minutes or until crisp. Let cool on pan on a wire rack.

This recipe courtesy of dietitian Jaclyn Pritchard.

Nutrients	
PER 2 TBSP (30 ML)	
Calories	55
Fat	2 g
Carbohydrate	9 g
Fiber	2 g
Protein	2 g

Pesto-Stuffed Tomatoes

*Pumpkin seeds are a
unique alternative to
pine nuts in the pesto
that fills these yummy
hors d'oeuvres.*

Tips

Green pumpkin seeds are
also known as pepitas. They
are often toasted to bring
out their nutty flavor. Be
sure to use hulled pumpkin
seeds in this recipe.

If you need a last-minute
appetizer, use purchased
basil pesto to make these
super-easy appetizers.

Variation

To give these appetizers
a cheesy twist, combine
half the pesto with ¼ cup
(60 mL) softened goat
cheese. Pipe into cored
tomatoes. Cover and
refrigerate the remaining
pesto for up to 2 days for
another use.

- **Food processor or blender**
- **Piping bag with medium-size round tip**

2	cloves garlic, minced	2
1 cup	packed fresh basil leaves	250 mL
⅓ cup	green pumpkin seeds (pepitas), toasted and cooled	75 mL
¼ tsp	salt	1 mL
¼ tsp	freshly ground black pepper	1 mL
3 tbsp	extra virgin olive oil	45 mL
24	cherry tomatoes, cored	24

1. In food processor, combine garlic, basil, pumpkin seeds, salt, pepper and oil; process until smooth.
2. Transfer pesto to piping bag and pipe into cherry tomatoes; do not overfill. Cover and refrigerate until chilled, for up to 4 hours.

This recipe courtesy of dietitian Heather McColl.

Nutrients
PER APPETIZER

Calories	30
Fat	3 g
Carbohydrate	1 g
Fiber	1 g
Protein	1 g

Spinach and Goat Cheese in Phyllo

Makes
60 appetizers

Phyllo dough is available in the freezer section of most supermarkets and makes a delicious wrap for these Greek-style appetizers.

Tips

Substitute 1 package (10 oz/300 g) fresh spinach for frozen and add to onion mixture; stir and cook for 4 to 5 minutes or until wilted. Cool and chop finely.

For best results, defrost phyllo pastry in the refrigerator overnight. This will preserve the quality of the pastry sheets.

- Preheat oven to 425°F (220°C)
- Rimmed baking sheet

Sauce

¼ cup	low-fat plain yogurt	60 mL
¼ cup	light sour cream	60 mL
¼ cup	finely diced seeded peeled cucumber	60 mL
1	clove garlic, minced	1

Filling

½ cup	olive oil, divided	125 mL
½ cup	finely chopped onion	125 mL
1	package (10 oz/300 g) frozen chopped spinach, thawed and squeezed to remove moisture	1
4 oz	crumbled soft goat cheese	125 g
1 tsp	salt	5 mL
¼ tsp	freshly ground black pepper	1 mL
¼ tsp	ground nutmeg	1 mL
1 lb	phyllo dough (about 20 sheets)	500 g

1. *Sauce:* In a small bowl, mix yogurt, sour cream, cucumber and garlic. Cover and chill for at least 1 hour before serving.

2. *Filling:* In a small skillet, heat 1 tbsp (15 mL) of the oil; cook onion, stirring, until softened. Remove from heat. Mix in spinach, cheese, salt, pepper and nutmeg until combined.

3. Place 1 sheet of phyllo on work surface, keeping remaining phyllo covered with a damp tea towel to prevent drying; brush sheet lightly with some of the oil and top with second sheet; brush with oil.

Nutrients
PER APPETIZER

Calories	48
Fat	2 g
Carbohydrate	5 g
Fiber	0 g
Protein	1 g

Whether you choose fresh or frozen vegetables, you are essentially getting the same nutrients. In fact, vegetables that have been frozen immediately after harvesting may contain more nutrients than those that must travel to reach you.

4. With a sharp knife or pizza cutter, cut phyllo lengthwise into 6 equal strips. Place about 1 tsp (5 mL) filling 1 inch (2.5 cm) from bottom end of strip; fold 1 corner to opposite side, forming a triangle that covers filling. Continue folding from side to side up entire length of strip. Place seam side down on baking sheet; repeat with remaining phyllo, oil and filling.

5. Brush tops lightly with oil. Cover with plastic wrap and refrigerate for up to 12 hours or freeze in airtight containers.

6. Bake triangles in preheated oven for about 10 minutes or until golden (frozen ones may take a little longer). Serve with sauce.

This recipe courtesy of chef Albert Cipryk and dietitian Cynthia Paul.

Homemade Salsa

This healthy salsa is great for dipping.

Tips

Tomatoes contain lycopene, a powerful natural antioxidant.

You'll need 2 to 3 limes for 3 tbsp (35 mL) juice.

Choose snacks with nutritional value, balanced in carbohydrates, fats and proteins where possible. Snacks prevent excessive hunger and help with weight management.

5	tomatoes, chopped	5
12	sprigs fresh cilantro, chopped	12
3 tbsp	freshly squeezed lime juice	45 mL
¾ tsp	salt	3 mL
½ tsp	garlic-infused olive oil	2 mL

1. In a bowl, whisk together tomatoes, cilantro, lime juice, salt and oil. Cover and refrigerate for at least 1 hour before serving.

Nutrients
PER SERVING

Calories	13
Fat	0 g
Carbohydrate	3 g
Fiber	1 g
Protein	1 g

Sardine and Pesto Spread

*Three simple ingredients
give big taste to this
chunky spread.*

Tips

Don't mash the sardines
too much, or you'll end
up with more of a paste
than a spread.

Try Mediterranean-style or
lemon-flavored sardines.

Serve with crudités, whole-
grain crackers or toasted
French baguette slices.

Sardines are an often
overlooked food. They are
a good choice for people
trying to increase their
intake of vitamin D, vitamin
B_{12} and health-promoting
omega-3 fats.

1	can (3½ oz/106 g) sardines, drained	1
2 tbsp	basil pesto	30 mL
1 tbsp	freshly squeezed lime juice	15 mL

1. In a small bowl, mash sardines with a fork. Stir in pesto
and lime juice until just blended.

This recipe courtesy of dietitian Claude Gamache.

Nutrients
PER 1 TBSP (15 ML)

Calories	37
Fat	3 g
Carbohydrate	1 g
Fiber	0 g
Protein	3 g

Piquant White Bean and Parsley Dip

Makes 1½ cups (375 mL)

If you're looking for a snack with some heat, this is it! This dip also makes a delicious spread for sandwiches, as an alternative to mayonnaise.

Tips

White kidney beans offer 8.6 to 9.9 g of fiber per ¾ cup (175 mL).

It's best to start by adding just one pepper to the dip, then you can add more to taste.

Spread some of this piquant dip inside a whole wheat pita pocket and fill it with roasted eggplant, zucchini, onions and peppers.

Variation

For Asian flair, add a few drops of sesame oil and garnish this dip with sesame seeds.

- **Food processor or blender**

2	green onions, coarsely chopped	2
2	cloves garlic, minced	2
1 to 2	jalapeño peppers, seeded and coarsely chopped	1 to 2
1	can (19 oz/540 mL) white kidney beans, drained and rinsed	1
½ cup	loosely packed chopped fresh parsley	125 mL
¼ cup	freshly squeezed lemon juice	60 mL
1 tbsp	canola oil	15 mL
1 tsp	ground cumin	5 mL

1. In food processor, combine green onions, garlic, jalapeños to taste, beans, parsley, lemon juice, oil and cumin; process until smooth.

2. Transfer to a bowl, cover and refrigerate for at least 1 hour, until chilled, or for up to 1 day.

This recipe courtesy of dietitian Mary Sue Waisman.

Nutrients	
PER 2 TBSP (30 ML)	
Calories	48
Fat	1 g
Carbohydrate	7 g
Fiber	3 g
Protein	2 g

Salmon Oasis

Makes 4 servings

This tasty combination of English muffins and salmon with a hint of zest makes a satisfying and delicious lunch.

Tip

Team this with a glass of skim milk and some fruit for a lunch that will go a long way toward meeting the daily requirement of many vitamins and minerals.

- **Preheat broiler**
- **Baking sheet, ungreased**

4	whole wheat English muffins	4
1	can (7½ oz/213 g) salmon, drained	1
¼ cup	light mayonnaise	60 mL
2 tbsp	finely chopped green onion	30 mL
2 tsp	freshly squeezed lemon juice	10 mL
½ tsp	curry powder	2 mL
¼ tsp	freshly ground black pepper	1 mL
8	green bell pepper strips	8
¾ cup	shredded part-skim mozzarella cheese	175 mL
	Paprika	

1. Split muffins in half and toast.
2. Combine salmon, mayonnaise, green onion, lemon juice, curry powder and pepper. Spread on muffin halves; top with green pepper and cheese. Sprinkle with paprika to taste. Place on ungreased baking sheet. Broil for about 3 minutes or just until cheese melts.

This recipe courtesy of Ellen Craig.

Nutrients
PER SERVING

Calories	154
Fat	6 g
Carbohydrate	13 g
Fiber	6 g
Protein	11 g

Tuna Salad Melt

This tuna mixture also makes a great filling for sandwiches, wraps and pita bread, and a great topping for salad greens. If desired, substitute salmon for the tuna.

Tips

One way to cut back on fat in tuna or egg salad is to use low-fat yogurt as a substitute for some of the mayonnaise.

Tuna is a good source of omega-3 fatty acids and a source of vitamin D.

Variations

Hot Tuna Salad Wrap: Fill flour tortillas with tuna mixture and shredded low-fat cheese. Fold up and microwave on High for 30 to 45 seconds or until cheese is melted.

Cold Tuna Salad Wrap: Add any shredded or grated vegetable to the tuna mixture. Roll in a tortilla and serve.

Nutrients
PER SERVING

Calories	208
Fat	6 g
Carbohydrate	24 g
Fiber	1 g
Protein	14 g

- **Preheat broiler**
- **Large baking sheet**

2	cans (6 oz/170 g) water-packed tuna, drained	2
¼ cup	finely chopped celery	60 mL
¼ cup	finely chopped sweet pickle or sweet relish	60 mL
¼ cup	finely chopped red or green bell pepper (optional)	60 mL
¼ cup	light mayonnaise	60 mL
2 tbsp	lower-fat plain yogurt	30 mL
1 tbsp	lemon juice or pickle juice	15 mL
1	French stick (baguette)	1
½ cup	shredded Cheddar cheese	125 mL

1. In a bowl, stir together tuna, celery, pickle, red pepper, if using, mayonnaise, yogurt and lemon juice. Blend well.

2. Slice French stick in half lengthwise. Cut each half into 4 equal portions, making 8 pieces; place on baking sheet. Toast under preheated broiler for 1 to 2 minutes or until golden.

3. Remove from broiler; spread tuna mixture evenly over each piece. Sprinkle with cheese. Broil for 2 to 3 minutes or until cheese is melted and golden.

This recipe courtesy of dietitian Bev Callaghan.

Rainbow Lettuce Wraps

Lettuce wraps are a fresh alternative to bread-based wraps. These are best assembled individually at the table.

Tips

You could also use cooled cooked cabbage leaves as the wraps.

Butter lettuce is a type of head lettuce that has, as the name implies, a smooth, buttery texture. Varieties of butter lettuce include Boston and Bibb.

Variation

Lean ground beef, pork or vegetarian ground round can be used in place of turkey.

1 lb	lean ground turkey or chicken	500 g
1 tbsp	grated gingerroot	15 mL
2 tsp	canola oil	10 mL
¾ cup	finely chopped red bell pepper	175 mL
¾ cup	finely chopped yellow bell pepper	175 mL
½ cup	finely chopped onion	125 mL
2	cloves garlic, minced	2
1	can (8 oz/227 mL) sliced water chestnuts, drained and chopped	1
¼ cup	hoisin sauce	60 mL
¾ tsp	Chinese five-spice powder	3 mL
¼ to ½ tsp	hot pepper flakes	1 to 2 mL
½ cup	shredded carrot	125 mL
1	head butter lettuce, leaves separated	1

1. In a large nonstick skillet, over medium heat, brown turkey and ginger, breaking up turkey with a spoon, for 5 to 6 minutes or until no longer pink. Transfer to a bowl and set aside.

2. In the same skillet, heat oil over medium heat. Sauté red pepper, yellow pepper and onion for 4 to 5 minutes or until vegetables are softened. Add garlic and sauté for 30 seconds. Return turkey to skillet and stir in water chestnuts, hoisin sauce, ¼ cup (60 mL) water, five-spice powder and hot pepper flakes to taste; cook, stirring often, for 3 to 4 minutes or until heated through. Transfer to a serving bowl.

3. Arrange carrot and lettuce leaves on a large platter and set out with the turkey mixture. Top each lettuce leaf with 2 tbsp (30 mL) of the turkey mixture, then carrot. Wrap lettuce to enclose filling.

This recipe courtesy of dietitian Heather McColl.

Nutrients PER 2 WRAPS	
Calories	69
Fat	3 g
Carbohydrate	5 g
Fiber	1 g
Protein	6 g

Chicken, Hummus and Sautéed Veggie Wraps

This recipe is easy to prepare and full of flavor.

Tips

This recipe can be fully prepared and refrigerated overnight for a great lunch, or its components can be stored separately in airtight containers for several days. Pop cold wraps in a toaster oven or microwave to heat through.

Serve with fruit salad for a delicious lunch.

1 lb	small boneless skinless chicken breasts	500 g
	Salt and freshly ground black pepper	
	Vegetable cooking spray	
1 tbsp	olive oil	15 mL
2	cloves garlic, minced	2
1	green bell pepper, julienned	1
1	red bell pepper, julienned	1
1	yellow bell pepper, julienned	1
1	onion, cut into thin strips	1
2	carrots, julienned	2
½ cup	water	125 mL
2 to 3 tsp	chili powder	10 to 15 mL
½ cup	Spicy Hummus (see recipe, opposite)	125 mL
4	10-inch (25 cm) whole wheat tortillas	4

1. Season chicken breasts with salt and pepper.

2. Heat a large skillet over medium heat. Spray with vegetable cooking spray. Cook chicken, turning once, for 5 minutes per side or until chicken is no longer pink inside and has reached an internal temperature of 170°F (77°C). Remove to a clean plate and let cool. Cut into strips.

3. In the same skillet, heat olive oil over medium-high heat. Sauté garlic, green, red and yellow peppers, onion and carrots, stirring frequently, until beginning to brown, about 5 minutes. Add water and chili powder; season to taste with salt and pepper. Reduce heat to medium and cook until vegetables are tender-crisp and water has evaporated, about 5 minutes.

4. Spread 2 tbsp (30 mL) Spicy Hummus up the middle of each tortilla. Top with chicken and vegetables. Roll up tortillas.

This recipe courtesy of Rena Hooey.

Nutrients
PER SERVING

Calories	366
Fat	7 g
Carbohydrate	51 g
Fiber	7 g
Protein	34 g

Spicy Hummus

Hummus makes a great sandwich spread for a vegetarian lunch, and is a delicious and nutritious between-meal snack with crackers, pitas or celery sticks. Most hummus recipes call for tahini, which is not always easy to find. This one, without tahini, is still excellent.

Tips

If the hummus is too thick for your taste, blend in a little water.

Hummus will keep for up to 1 week in the refrigerator.

Serve hummus in a hollowed-out red pepper for a nice presentation when entertaining.

- **Blender or food processor**

1	can (19 oz/540 mL) chickpeas, drained and rinsed (about 2 cups/500 mL)	1
2	cloves garlic	2
1/4 tsp	ground cumin	1 mL
1/4 tsp	ground coriander	1 mL
1/4 tsp	hot pepper sauce	1 mL
1 tbsp	freshly squeezed lemon juice	15 mL

1. In blender, on medium speed, blend chickpeas, garlic, cumin, coriander and hot pepper sauce for 30 seconds or until finely chopped. Add lemon juice and blend until smooth.

Nutrients
PER SERVING

Calories	88
Fat	1 g
Carbohydrate	17 g
Fiber	3 g
Protein	4 g

Bulgur and Vegetable Lettuce Wraps

Makes about 2 cups (500 mL) filling

These delicious vegetarian appetizers are filled with fresh flavor and color.

Tips

For guaranteed success with an herb garden, start by growing mint. It grows well in most climates and grows wild in many parts of North America.

Add a wedge of low-fat cheese and a piece of fresh fruit to turn this snack into a wholesome lunch.

Variations

Use black beans or kidney beans instead of chickpeas.

Add some heat to the mixture with minced jalapeño or a few drops of hot pepper sauce.

¾ cup	bulgur	175 mL
¾ cup	warm water	175 mL
1 cup	diced tomatoes	250 mL
½ cup	cooked or canned chickpeas, drained and rinsed	125 mL
¼ cup	chopped fresh parsley	60 mL
2 tbsp	chopped green onion	30 mL
2 tbsp	chopped red onion	30 mL
1 tbsp	chopped fresh mint	15 mL
2 tbsp	canola oil	30 mL
1 tbsp	freshly squeezed lemon juice	15 mL
¼ tsp	salt	1 mL
½ tsp	freshly ground black pepper	2 mL
1	head butter lettuce, leaves separated	1

1. In a large bowl, combine bulgur and warm water. Let stand for 30 minutes, until bulgur is softened and liquid is absorbed.

2. Add tomatoes, chickpeas, parsley, green onion, red onion, mint, oil, lemon juice, salt and pepper. Stir well to combine.

3. Top each lettuce leaf with 2 tbsp (30 mL) bulgur mixture. Wrap lettuce to enclose filling.

This recipe courtesy of dietitian Leila Smaily.

Nutrients
PER 2 WRAPS

Calories	50
Fat	2 g
Carbohydrate	7 g
Fiber	1 g
Protein	2 g

Big-Batch Whole Wheat Pizza Dough

Makes enough dough for two 12- to 15-inch (30 to 38 cm) pizza crusts

A homemade crust, when you have time to prepare it, makes a huge difference to the taste of your pizza and provides added nutrition. It seems like a long process, but it is relatively easy. Try this dough with Ham and Pineapple Pizza (page 172), or create your own pizza parlor special!

Tip

If you do not have an electric mixer with a dough hook, you can use a food processor.

- **Electric mixer with dough hook**

2	packages (each ¼ oz/7 g) instant yeast	2
2 cups	whole wheat flour	500 mL
1 cup	all-purpose flour	250 mL
1 tsp	salt	5 mL
½ tsp	granulated sugar	2 mL
1½ cups	lukewarm water	375 mL
½ tsp	olive oil	2 mL

1. In the mixer bowl, combine yeast, whole wheat flour, all-purpose flour, salt and sugar. Attach dough hook and mixer bowl to mixer. With mixer running on low speed, gradually add water; knead until dough is smooth and elastic, about 10 minutes. Turn mixer off and pour oil down side of bowl. Set to low speed for 15 seconds to coat inside of bowl and cover dough lightly with oil. Remove mixer bowl and cover loosely with plastic wrap.

2. Let rise in a warm, draft-free place until doubled in bulk, about 2 hours.

3. Punch down dough and cut in half to make two balls. Place each ball in an airtight freezer bag and store for up to 3 months, or roll out for immediate usage.

4. To roll out, place dough ball on a floured work surface and form into a circle. Roll out until dough reaches a 12- to 15-inch (30 to 38 cm) diameter. Pierce dough with a fork before adding toppings.

This recipe courtesy of Eileen Campbell.

Nutrients
PER ⅙ PIZZA CRUST

Calories	129
Fat	1 g
Carbohydrate	27 g
Fiber	4 g
Protein	5 g

Ham and Pineapple Pizza

A homemade pizza can be a delicious and nutritious lunch or dinner meal.

Tip

If you don't have time to make the dough, you can use a purchased pizza crust.

Variation

For a special treat, substitute diced mango for the pineapple and diced cooked chicken for the ham.

- **Preheat oven to 375°F (190°C)**
- **12-inch (30 cm) pizza pan, lightly greased**

1/2	recipe Big-Batch Whole Wheat Pizza Dough (page 171)	1/2
1/2	can (7 1/2 oz/213 mL) pizza sauce	1/2
1/2 cup	diced lean ham	125 mL
1/2 cup	diced fresh pineapple	125 mL
1 cup	shredded part-skim mozzarella	250 mL

1. Roll out dough to a 12-inch (30 cm) diameter and fit into prepared pan. Spread pizza sauce evenly over crust to within 1/2 inch (1 cm) of edge. Sprinkle evenly with ham and pineapple. Top with cheese.

2. Bake in preheated oven for 10 to 12 minutes or until cheese is melted and starting to brown and crust is golden and crisp.

This recipe courtesy of dietitian Donna Bottrell.

Nutrients PER SERVING	
Calories	154
Fat	2 g
Carbohydrate	23 g
Fiber	4 g
Protein	13 g

Soups

My Mother's Borscht

This dish is a must for anyone who loves beets. Borscht can be served hot or cold.

Tips

Make sure to garnish as suggested — the sour cream and fresh dill add a special touch.

If you choose to prepare this recipe in a slow cooker instead of on the stovetop, do not precook the beets. Also, wait to add the beet greens and stems until about 20 minutes before cooking is complete, and finish cooking on High.

Variation

Besides the vegetables listed in the recipe, you can use fresh tomatoes, cabbage, spinach and peppers, virtually cleaning out the vegetable crisper.

6	beets, with their green tops	6
2 cups	chopped onions	500 mL
1½ cups	chopped carrots	375 mL
1 cup	chopped celery	250 mL
2	cloves garlic, chopped	2
1	can (19 oz/540 mL) diced tomatoes (about 2⅓ cups/575 mL)	1
2 cups	chopped peeled potatoes	500 mL
2 cups	chicken broth or water	500 mL
1 tbsp	white vinegar	15 mL
1 tbsp	Worcestershire sauce	15 mL
1 tsp	chopped fresh dill (optional)	5 mL
	Hot pepper sauce	
	Light sour cream and chopped fresh dill	

1. Cut beet tops about 1 inch (2.5 cm) from beets. Wash thoroughly and drain. Coarsely chop greens and stems; set aside.

2. In a large covered saucepan, over medium-high heat, cook unpeeled beets in lots of boiling water. Cook for 20 to 30 minutes or until fork-tender. Cool quickly by running cold water over the beets; slip skins off under running water. Chop beets into ½-inch (1 cm) cubes and return to saucepan. Add beet greens and stems, onions, carrots, celery, garlic, tomatoes, potatoes, broth, vinegar, Worcestershire sauce, dill and hot pepper sauce to taste. Cover and cook over medium heat for 1 to 1½ hours or until vegetables are just tender.

3. Ladle into bowls and garnish with sour cream and dill.

This recipe courtesy of Madeleine Mitchell.

Nutrients
PER SERVING

Calories	81
Fat	0 g
Carbohydrate	18 g
Fiber	3 g
Protein	3 g

Cream of Broccoli Soup

This is a fast and easy soup for a chilly day. It tastes decadent too!

Tips

You can also use leftover cooked vegetables for this soup. Carrots, cauliflower or a combination work well.

Chromium is found in small amounts in a variety of foods, including broccoli.

• Blender

1	large head broccoli, chopped	1
1	small onion, chopped	1
2 cups	vegetable broth	500 mL
1	can (14 oz or 370 mL) evaporated milk	1
½ tsp	dried dillweed	2 mL
	Salt and freshly ground black pepper	
¼ cup	shredded Cheddar, freshly grated Parmesan or shredded Swiss cheese (optional)	60 mL

1. In a large saucepan, over medium heat, combine broccoli, onion and broth. Cover and bring to a boil. Reduce heat and simmer until vegetables are cooked, about 10 minutes. Remove from heat.

2. Working in batches, transfer soup to blender and purée on high speed until smooth.

3. Return soup to saucepan and add evaporated milk and dill. Heat over low heat (do not boil or milk could curdle). Season with salt and pepper to taste. Stir in cheese, if desired.

This recipe courtesy of dietitian Lisa Diamond.

Nutrients
PER SERVING

Calories	124
Fat	2 g
Carbohydrate	18 g
Fiber	3 g
Protein	10 g

Barley Vegetable Soup

When the weather's cold, a big pot of soup simmering on the stove warms the heart as well as the hearth. Whole-grain barley gives this soup its robust flavor.

Tips

If you prefer your vegetables sautéed in oil, add 1 tbsp (15 mL) vegetable oil to the saucepan and heat over medium heat, then sauté the celery, onion and carrot before adding the tomatoes, broth, barley and pepper. But keep in mind that doing this will affect the nutrient analysis, since you are adding fat to the recipe.

A piece of low-fat cheese and some crusty bread will make this a satisfying lunch.

1	can (19 oz/540 mL) diced tomatoes (about 2⅓ cups/575 mL)	1
6 cups	chicken broth	1.5 L
½ cup	diced celery	125 mL
½ cup	diced onion	125 mL
½ cup	diced carrot	125 mL
½ cup	barley	125 mL
	Freshly ground black pepper	

1. In a large saucepan, over medium heat, combine tomatoes, broth, celery, onion, carrot, barley and pepper to taste; bring to a boil. Reduce heat, cover and simmer for 1 hour or until barley is soft.

This recipe courtesy of dietitian Claude Gamache.

Nutrients
PER SERVING

Calories	78
Fat	0 g
Carbohydrate	15 g
Fiber	2 g
Protein	3 g

Green Pea and Tarragon Soup

Makes 6 servings

The flavors in this soup are a winning combination, especially if you can find fresh peas. Fresh tarragon is a key ingredient.

Tips

The green peas in this soup provide an excellent source of fiber.

Be sure not to brown the shallots or you will have unpleasant brown bits in your soup.

This soup may be strained after it is puréed. The resulting soup will be very thin, and much of the fibrous pea matter will be removed.

This soup makes a pleasant first course before a beef- or pork-based dinner.

Star anise has a pleasant licorice flavor similar to anise. It is the seed of a Chinese evergreen tree and is one of the ingredients in Chinese five-spice powder.

Nutrients PER SERVING	
Calories	101
Fat	1 g
Carbohydrate	16 g
Fiber	6 g
Protein	7 g

- **Food processor, blender or immersion blender**

1 tsp	canola oil	5 mL
¼ cup	finely chopped shallots	60 mL
¼ cup	loosely packed chopped fresh tarragon	60 mL
1	star anise pod	1
4 cups	fresh or frozen green peas (thawed if frozen)	1 L
4 cups	reduced-sodium chicken broth	1 L
½ tsp	freshly ground white pepper	2 mL
½ tsp	salt (optional)	2 mL

1. In a large pot, heat oil over medium heat. Sauté shallots for about 3 minutes or until softened, being careful not to brown them. Add tarragon and sauté for 30 seconds. Add star anise, peas and broth; bring to boil. Reduce heat and simmer for about 20 minutes or until peas are very tender. Discard star anise.

2. Working in batches, transfer soup to food processor (or use immersion blender in pot) and purée until smooth. Return soup to pot (if necessary) and stir in white pepper and salt (if using).

This recipe courtesy of dietitian Mary Sue Waisman.

Spinach Soup

This quick, easy soup is a delicious way to add spinach to your day.

Tips

Spinach is a source of soluble fiber.

Chopping the spinach before adding it to the pot makes it easier to eat and disperses the color throughout the soup more evenly.

Variation

Add leftover chopped cooked chicken or other chopped vegetables to make it a more complete meal.

1 tbsp	canola oil	15 mL
1 cup	chopped onion	250 mL
2	cloves garlic, minced	2
1	package (10 oz/300 g) baby spinach, roughly chopped	1
4 cups	reduced-sodium chicken broth	1 L
1/2 cup	peperini, orzo or other tiny pasta	125 mL
	Freshly ground black pepper	
1/4 cup	freshly grated Parmesan cheese	60 mL

1. In a large pot, heat oil over medium heat. Sauté onion for 3 to 4 minutes or until softened. Add garlic and sauté for 30 seconds. Add spinach and cook, stirring, for 2 to 3 minutes or until spinach is tender and reduced in volume by at least half.

2. Add broth, increase heat to high and bring to a boil. Stir in pasta, reduce heat and simmer for 5 to 7 minutes or until pasta is tender. Ladle into bowls, sprinkle with pepper to taste and garnish with cheese.

This recipe courtesy of Carmelina Salomone.

If you're feeling confident about your cooking skills, you can make a unique and pleasant finish for this soup. As the soup is cooking, in a small bowl, combine 1 beaten egg and 1 tbsp (15 mL) of the Parmesan, whisking until cheese is incorporated. Gradually whisk in 2 tbsp (30 mL) hot broth from the soup. Remove soup from the heat and very, very gradually add the egg mixture to the pot, stirring as you add it. Ladle into bowls and sprinkle with the remaining cheese. The resulting broth will be velvety in texture.

Note: It's important to add a bit of soup to the egg mixture so that the temperature of the egg mixture is close to that of the soup. Otherwise, the heat of the soup will scramble the egg when you add it.

Nutrients
PER SERVING

Calories	122
Fat	4 g
Carbohydrate	16 g
Fiber	2 g
Protein	7 g

Country Lentil Soup

This hearty soup can be satisfying for lunch or dinner. Soups made with legumes are sources of fiber.

Tip

If you prefer, when puréeing soups you can use an immersion blender and blend the soup right in the pot. This will save you some cleanup time, but the result will be less smooth.

Variations

Substitute green lentils, well rinsed and drained, canned chickpeas or white kidney beans for the red lentils. Decrease the simmering time to 15 minutes if using canned legumes.

To make this a heartier soup, add 1 cup (250 mL) of diced cooked lean ham after puréeing.

- **Blender**

1 tbsp	vegetable oil	15 mL
1 cup	diced onion	250 mL
½ cup	diced carrot	125 mL
½ cup	diced celery	125 mL
4 cups	vegetable or chicken broth	1 L
1 cup	dried red lentils, well rinsed	250 mL
¼ tsp	dried thyme	1 mL
	Salt and freshly ground black pepper	
½ cup	chopped fresh flat-leaf parsley	125 mL

1. In a large saucepan, heat oil over medium heat. Sauté onion, carrot and celery until softened, about 5 minutes. Add broth, lentils and thyme; bring to a boil. Reduce heat, cover and simmer for 20 minutes or until lentils are soft. Remove from heat.

2. Working in batches, transfer soup to blender. Purée on high speed until creamy. Add up to 1 cup (250 mL) water if purée is too thick. Season with salt and pepper to taste. Return to saucepan to reheat, if necessary.

3. Ladle into bowls and garnish with parsley.

This recipe courtesy of Eileen Campbell.

Nutrients
PER SERVING

Calories	117
Fat	2 g
Carbohydrate	19 g
Fiber	4 g
Protein	4 g

Egg Lemon Soup

This is a popular soup in Greece, where the Greek word avgolemeno *names the two staple ingredients, egg and lemon.*

6 cups	vegetable or chicken broth	1.5 L
1 cup	long-grain converted rice	250 mL
3	eggs, beaten	3
	Juice of 2 lemons	
	Salt and freshly ground black pepper	
2 cups	diced cooked chicken	500 mL
	Additional freshly squeezed lemon juice	

1. In a medium, heavy-bottomed pot, bring chicken broth and rice to a boil over high heat. Reduce heat to medium-low and simmer for 20 minutes or until rice is tender. Leave pot on burner, but turn off heat.

2. Meanwhile, in a medium bowl, using an electric mixer on high, beat together eggs and lemon juice until blended. While beating on high, slowly pour 1 ladleful of broth mixture into egg mixture (to prevent eggs from curdling). In same manner, add 2 more ladlefuls of broth mixture to egg mixture. Briskly whisk egg mixture into remaining broth mixture in pot (soup will have a creamy, cloudy appearance). Season to taste with salt and pepper.

3. Stir in chicken. If necessary, gently simmer soup over medium-low heat, stirring occasionally, until heated through. Stir in lemon juice to taste.

Nutrients
PER SERVING

Calories	241
Fat	6 g
Carbohydrate	29 g
Fiber	1 g
Protein	16 g

Hot and Sour Chicken Soup

Makes 6 servings

Impress friends and family with your own version of this Chinese classic.

Tips

Use thin green or red chiles or Thai finger chiles in this recipe rather than jalapeño chiles. If using a fresh chile pepper, wash your hands thoroughly after chopping.

The tofu, chicken and egg whites in this soup combine to make a good source of protein.

6	dried Chinese mushrooms	6
5	cups chicken broth	1.25 L
2 cups	shredded cooked chicken (7 oz/200 g)	500 mL
1 tbsp	finely chopped gingerroot	15 mL
1	chile pepper, chopped (or $\frac{1}{2}$ tsp/2 mL hot pepper flakes)	1
1 cup	diced firm tofu	250 mL
2 tbsp	white wine vinegar	30 mL
1 tbsp	sodium-reduced soy sauce	15 mL
1 tbsp	dry sherry	15 mL
1 tbsp	cornstarch	15 mL
1 tbsp	cold water	15 mL
3	egg whites, lightly beaten	3
2	shallots, thinly sliced (optional)	2

1. Cover Chinese mushrooms with hot water and soak for 10 minutes. Drain, discard stems and slice caps.

2. In a large saucepan, bring broth to a boil; add mushrooms, chicken, gingerroot and chile pepper. Reduce heat and simmer, covered, for 5 minutes. Add tofu, vinegar, soy sauce and sherry; simmer for 2 minutes.

3. Stir cornstarch with water until smooth; gradually stir into soup and simmer for 2 to 3 minutes or until thickened slightly. Remove from heat; immediately swirl egg whites through soup. Garnish with shallots, if desired.

This recipe courtesy of chef Raymond Colliver and dietitian Dani Flowerday.

Nutrients
PER SERVING

Calories	145
Fat	5 g
Carbohydrate	6 g
Fiber	1 g
Protein	18 g

Curried Coconut Chicken Soup

Makes 8 servings

This Thai favorite is easy to make at home. For a less spicy dish, reduce the amount of curry paste, or leave it out, and cut back on the amount of ginger.

Tips

Puréed ginger, available in jars from your grocery store, will save a few minutes in preparation time.

For a more authentic flavor, use wild lime leaves, when available, instead of grated zest. Substitute 3 leaves for the zest of 1 lime.

1	can (14 oz/398 mL) light coconut milk	1
1 tsp	red curry paste	5 mL
2 cups	reduced-sodium chicken broth	500 mL
3	stalks lemongrass, split in half lengthwise (or 1 tsp/5 mL finely grated lemon zest)	3
2	boneless skinless chicken breasts (about 8 oz/250 g total), cut into thin strips	2
¼ cup	finely grated gingerroot	60 mL
1 tbsp	fish sauce (approx.)	15 mL
1	lime	1
2 cups	baby spinach leaves	500 mL
1	green onion, chopped	1
½ cup	chopped fresh cilantro	125 mL

1. Take ½ cup (125 mL) from the top layer of coconut milk and place in a large saucepan over medium heat. Heat to bubbling, then stir in red curry paste. Reduce heat and simmer for 5 minutes. Add remaining coconut milk and broth; increase heat to medium and bring to a boil. Add lemongrass, chicken, ginger and fish sauce; return to a boil. Reduce heat and simmer, uncovered, until chicken is cooked through, about 8 minutes.

2. Grate zest from the lime, then squeeze the juice. Add lime zest, 1 tbsp (15 mL) lime juice and baby spinach to the soup; simmer for 5 minutes. Remove lemongrass and discard. Taste and add lime juice and fish sauce, if desired.

3. Ladle into bowls and garnish with green onion and cilantro.

This recipe courtesy of Eileen Campbell.

Nutrients
PER SERVING

Calories	130
Fat	6 g
Carbohydrate	7 g
Fiber	1 g
Protein	12 g

Chicken and Corn Chowder

Makes 9 servings

The evaporated milk in this delicious, creamy soup gives it a richness that suggests it is higher in fat than it actually is. The addition of sweet potato and red pepper helps increase your intake of beta carotene and vitamin C.

Variation

This soup works just as well without the chicken. Try replacing it with drained canned clams for variety. With clams, a little hot pepper sauce makes a nice addition.

1 tbsp	non-hydrogenated margarine	15 mL
1 cup	finely chopped onion	250 mL
1 cup	diced celery	250 mL
½ cup	finely chopped red bell pepper	125 mL
1	boneless skinless chicken breast (about 4 oz/125 g), cubed	1
4 cups	reduced-sodium chicken broth	1 L
1 cup	diced peeled sweet potato	250 mL
1 cup	frozen corn kernels, thawed	250 mL
1	can (14 oz or 370 mL) 2% evaporated milk	1
1 tbsp	chopped fresh parsley	15 mL

1. In a large saucepan, melt margarine over medium heat. Sauté onion, celery and red pepper until softened, about 5 minutes.
2. Add chicken, broth, sweet potato and corn; bring to a boil. Reduce heat, cover and simmer for 25 minutes or until chicken and potatoes are cooked through. Add evaporated milk and parsley; heat over low heat (do not boil or milk will curdle).

This recipe courtesy of Eileen Campbell.

Nutrients
PER SERVING

Calories	118
Fat	3 g
Carbohydrate	14 g
Fiber	1 g
Protein	10 g

Hamburger Soup

This hearty, family-style soup is perfect for a cold-weather dinner or après-ski. The addition of pasta or barley (see variation, below) makes it a complete meal. The recipe makes a large quantity, but the soup freezes well.

Tip

For variety, replace the kidney beans with about 2 cups (500 mL) of a medley of mixed frozen beans. These assortments usually include chickpeas, kidney, black, romano and white (navy) beans.

Variation

For a more robust meal, add uncooked pasta or barley (about ½ cup/125 mL) to this soup. Add barley with vegetables and cook for 35 minutes. If using pasta, add with zucchini and cook for 10 minutes.

Nutrients		
PER SERVING		
Calories		145
Fat		5 g
Carbohydrate		15 g
Fiber		4 g
Protein		11 g

1 lb	lean ground beef	500 g
1	can (28 oz/796 mL) tomatoes	1
1	can (19 oz/540 mL) kidney beans, drained and rinsed	1
1	can (10 oz/284 mL) condensed tomato soup	1
5 cups	water	1.25 L
1	onion, chopped	1
1	carrot, chopped	1
½ cup	chopped celery	125 mL
½ cup	sliced mushrooms	125 mL
1 tsp	Worcestershire sauce	5 mL
¼ tsp	hot pepper sauce	1 mL
¼ tsp	freshly ground black pepper	1 mL
2	small zucchini, chopped	2

1. In a large stockpot over medium heat, brown beef until crumbly; drain fat. Add tomatoes, kidney beans, tomato soup, water, onion, carrot, celery, mushrooms and seasonings; bring to a boil. Reduce heat and simmer, covered, for about 35 minutes. Add zucchini. Simmer for 10 minutes longer.

This recipe courtesy of Paula Worton.

Salads

Citrus Fennel Slaw

The fennel and citrus combination is a natural in this crunchy twist on coleslaw.

Tips

Fresh fennel is reasonably new to North American cuisine, though it's been used extensively in Mediterranean cooking for centuries. It has a mild licorice flavor. The bulb is delicious used in salads, soups and stews. The frond, though beautiful, is rarely used in cooking.

To get thin, even slices, use a mandoline to cut the fennel bulb.

Instead of serving on top of greens on individual plates, you can also simply pass the slaw.

Variation

Substitute toasted unsalted sunflower seeds for the pine nuts.

1	large fennel bulb	1
¼	red onion, very thinly sliced	¼
	Grated zest and juice of 1 lemon	
	Grated zest of 1 orange	
2 tbsp	freshly squeezed orange juice	30 mL
1 tbsp	canola oil	15 mL
Pinch	salt	Pinch
	Freshly ground black pepper	
6 cups	mesclun mix	1.5 L
3 tbsp	toasted pine nuts	45 mL

1. Remove the stalks and tough outer leaves of the fennel bulb and discard. Cut bulb in half lengthwise and trim out core. Cut bulb crosswise into very thin slices.

2. Place fennel slices and red onion in a large bowl. Stir in lemon zest, lemon juice, orange zest and orange juice. Drizzle with oil and sprinkle with salt and pepper to taste.

3. Divide mesclun mix evenly among six small plates. Mound one-sixth of the fennel slaw on each plate and garnish with pine nuts.

This recipe courtesy of dietitian Jaclyn Pritchard.

Nutrients
PER SERVING

Calories	85
Fat	5 g
Carbohydrate	9 g
Fiber	3 g
Protein	2 g

Beet, Orange and Jicama Salad

Jicama is a crunchy, slightly sweet vegetable that tastes like a cross between a water chestnut and an apple. It adds a delicious crunch to this salad. If you can't find it at your supermarket, substitute an equal quantity of fresh fennel.

Tip

Broaden your culinary horizons — and your nutrient intake — by trying a new vegetable each week. How about jicama, celeriac, rapini, kohlrabi or Swiss chard?

1	can (14 oz/398 mL) sliced beets, drained	1
2	large navel oranges, peeled and cut into ¼-inch (0.5 cm) slices	2
½ cup	thinly sliced sweet white onion	125 mL
½ cup	julienned jicama	125 mL

Dressing

2 tbsp	balsamic vinegar	30 mL
1 tbsp	orange juice	15 mL
1 tbsp	olive oil	15 mL
⅛ tsp	salt	0.5 mL
	Freshly ground black pepper	
1 tbsp	chopped fresh parsley (optional)	15 mL

1. In a medium bowl, combine beets, oranges, onion and jicama. Set aside.

2. *Dressing:* In a small bowl, whisk together vinegar, orange juice, olive oil, salt and pepper to taste. Add to beet mixture; toss gently. Chill. Sprinkle with parsley, if using, just before serving.

This recipe courtesy of dietitian Bev Callaghan.

Nutrients
PER SERVING

Calories	71
Fat	2 g
Carbohydrate	12 g
Fiber	3 g
Protein	1 g

Cucumber Watermelon Salad

This salad is vibrant in color, crisp in texture and bursting with flavor — perfect for a hot summer day.

Tip

This salad becomes very liquidy if left overnight, but there likely won't be any leftovers to worry about!

Variation

For a twist, drizzle with 1 tbsp (15 mL) balsamic vinegar.

½	seedless watermelon, rind removed, flesh cut into 1-inch (2.5 cm) chunks (4 to 6 cups/1 to 1.5 L)	½
1	English cucumber, quartered lengthwise, seeds removed, cut into ¼-inch (0.5 cm) slices	1
1 tbsp	canola or extra virgin olive oil	15 mL
½ cup	finely chopped fresh basil	125 mL
½ cup	crumbled feta cheese	125 mL

1. In a large bowl, combine watermelon and cucumber. Drizzle with oil. Add basil and cheese; gently toss to combine.

This recipe courtesy of Brendine Partyka.

Nutrients
PER SERVING

Calories	69
Fat	4 g
Carbohydrate	8 g
Fiber	1 g
Protein	2 g

Greens with Strawberries

Be creative when purchasing greens for this tasty salad. Try different combinations of red leaf lettuce, pungent arugula, peppery watercress and sharp radicchio, as well as Bibb and iceberg lettuce. Or add a handful or two of mesclun mix to torn romaine.

Tips

The strawberries in this recipe are put to an unusual use — in the dressing. Combined with the greens, they are a great source of folate and vitamin C.

If desired, replace the strawberries with drained canned mandarin oranges.

When using raw sprouts, rinse and dry thoroughly before using to ensure that any harmful bacteria don't proliferate.

4 cups	assorted lettuce, torn into bite-size pieces	1 L
½ cup	sliced red onion	125 mL
½ cup	alfalfa sprouts	125 mL
Dressing		
¼ cup	orange juice	60 mL
1 tbsp	lemon juice	15 mL
1 tbsp	chopped fresh mint	15 mL
1 tsp	granulated sugar	5 mL
½ tsp	grated orange zest	2 mL
¼ tsp	grated lemon zest	1 mL
1 cup	sliced fresh strawberries	250 mL

1. In a salad bowl, combine lettuce, onion and sprouts; cover and refrigerate.

2. *Dressing:* Combine orange and lemon juices, mint, sugar and orange and lemon zest. Pour over sliced strawberries; cover and refrigerate.

3. Just before serving, pour strawberry mixture over salad greens; toss gently.

This recipe courtesy of Janice McDowell.

Nutrients
PER SERVING

Calories	23
Fat	0 g
Carbohydrate	5 g
Fiber	1 g
Protein	1 g

Spinach and Goat Cheese Salad

Makes 8 servings

This delicious salad is a healthy choice as a side salad, or add a piece of chicken breast to make it a meal.

Tips

The vinaigrette makes 1 cup (250 mL), but you only need ⅓ cup (75 mL) for 8 servings. Place the remainder in a jar, cover and refrigerate for up to 1 week.

Topped with slices of grilled chicken, this salad makes a terrific main course.

- **Blender or food processor**

8 cups	baby spinach	2 L
1	can (10 oz/284 mL) juice-packed mandarin orange segments, drained	1
½	large red onion, finely diced	½
2 oz	goat cheese, crumbled	60 g
¼ cup	honey-roasted almonds	60 mL
¼ cup	dried cranberries	60 mL

Dressing

¾ cup	thawed frozen raspberries	175 mL
2 tbsp	granulated sugar	30 mL
2 tbsp	canola oil	30 mL
4 tsp	raspberry-flavored vinegar	20 mL
1 tsp	poppy seeds	5 mL

1. In a large bowl, combine spinach, oranges, red onion, goat cheese, almonds and cranberries.

2. *Dressing:* In blender, combine raspberries, sugar, 3 tbsp (45 mL) water, oil and vinegar; blend until smooth. Pour into a small bowl and stir in poppy seeds.

3. Pour ⅓ cup (75 mL) of the dressing over the salad and toss to coat; reserve the remainder for another use.

This recipe courtesy of dietitian Jessica Kelly.

Nutrients
PER SERVING

Calories	97
Fat	5 g
Carbohydrate	11 g
Fiber	2 g
Protein	3 g

Tomato Mozzarella Salad

Makes 8 servings

Eating healthy is just this easy and tasty.

Tips

When tomatoes are in season, there's no better way to enjoy them than in this simple, delicious salad with an Italian flair. If desired, substitute fresh or Buffalo mozzarella for the part-skim version, but be aware that the Fat content will go up.

To ripen tomatoes, place them in a brown paper bag with an apple or a pear. These fruits give off ethylene dioxide, which causes the tomatoes to ripen.

Vinaigrette

¼ cup	canola or olive oil	60 mL
2 tbsp	vinegar	30 mL
1 tbsp	chopped fresh parsley	15 mL
2 tsp	Dijon mustard	10 mL
1 tsp	granulated sugar	5 mL
2	cloves garlic, minced	2
½ tsp	dried basil	2 mL
½ tsp	freshly ground black pepper	2 mL
¼ tsp	salt	1 mL
2 tbsp	water	30 mL

Salad

3	large tomatoes, preferably beefsteak	3
16	romaine or Boston lettuce leaves	16
½ cup	cubed part-skim mozzarella cheese	125 mL
6	green onions, sliced	6

1. *Vinaigrette:* In a jar with tight-fitting lid, whisk together oil, vinegar, parsley, mustard, sugar, garlic, basil, pepper, salt and water; chill. Shake before using.

2. *Salad:* Cut tomatoes in half; cut each half crosswise into slices. Arrange 2 lettuce leaves on each of eight salad plates. Arrange tomato slices on lettuce; sprinkle with cheese and green onion.

3. At serving time, pour vinaigrette over each salad.

This recipe courtesy of chef Yvonne C. Levert and dietitian Nanette Porter-MacDonald.

Nutrients
PER SERVING

Calories	106
Fat	8 g
Carbohydrate	6 g
Fiber	1 g
Protein	3 g

Herbed Green Potato Salad

Take this fresh, flavorful, healthy potato salad along to your next summertime barbecue and impress your neighbors. It's a great alternative to heavy, mayonnaise-based potato salad.

Tips

Grow your own herbs in pots on your patio or in your backyard. In the winter, you can bring them inside and keep them going on a sunny windowsill. That way, you'll always have fresh herbs at your fingertips.

New potatoes are sometimes called baby potatoes or creamer potatoes. They are immature potatoes that are harvested before the rest of the potato crop. They come in a variety of colors, are waxy in texture and have a paper-thin skin that generally does not need to be removed.

2 lbs	tiny new potatoes (unpeeled)	1 kg
2 tbsp	white wine vinegar	30 mL
2	cloves garlic, minced	2
2 tbsp	finely chopped fresh parsley	30 mL
2 tbsp	finely snipped fresh chives	30 mL
2 tbsp	finely snipped fresh dill	30 mL
2 tbsp	finely minced fresh sage	30 mL
1 tsp	freshly ground black pepper	5 mL
Pinch	salt	Pinch
2 tbsp	canola or olive oil	30 mL
2 tbsp	freshly squeezed lemon juice or orange juice	30 mL
½ cup	cooked green peas	125 mL

1. Place potatoes in a medium saucepan and add enough cold water to cover. Bring to a boil over medium-high heat; reduce heat and boil gently for 15 to 20 minutes or until just tender. Drain and let cool slightly. Cut potatoes in half and transfer to a bowl. Add vinegar, toss and set aside for 30 minutes.

2. In a small bowl, combine garlic, parsley, chives, dill, sage, pepper, salt, oil and lemon juice. Pour over potatoes and stir gently to coat. Stir in peas.

This recipe courtesy of dietitian Adam Hudson.

Nutrients
PER SERVING

Calories	165
Fat	5 g
Carbohydrate	28 g
Fiber	3 g
Protein	3 g

Best Bean Salad

Canned beans are a time saver and work very well in this dish.

Tips

Be sure to wash cilantro thoroughly, as it often contains a lot of grit.

Add half an egg salad sandwich and a glass of milk for a satisfying lunch.

2	large tomatoes, chopped	2
1	can (19 oz/540 mL) mixed bean medley, drained and rinsed	1
¼ cup	finely sliced red onion	60 mL
¼ cup	chopped fresh cilantro	60 mL
2 tbsp	chopped fresh basil	30 mL

Dressing

1	clove garlic, minced	1
¼ tsp	hot pepper flakes	1 mL
¼ tsp	freshly ground black pepper	1 mL
Pinch	salt	Pinch
1½ tbsp	extra virgin olive oil	22 mL
2 tsp	balsamic vinegar	10 mL
1 tsp	freshly squeezed lemon juice	5 mL

1. In a medium bowl, combine tomatoes, bean medley, red onion, cilantro and basil.

2. *Dressing:* In a small bowl, whisk together garlic, hot pepper flakes, black pepper, salt, oil, vinegar and lemon juice.

3. Pour dressing over bean mixture and toss gently to coat. Cover and refrigerate for at least 1 hour, until chilled, or for up to 1 day.

This recipe courtesy of dietitian Lucia Weiler.

Nutrients
PER SERVING

Calories	143
Fat	4 g
Carbohydrate	21 g
Fiber	6 g
Protein	7 g

Vegetable Quinoa Salad

Quinoa can be used in any recipe in which you would use rice, and can be served hot or cold. It is easy to cook.

Tips

If you are not a fan of the strong flavors of hot pepper and/or lavender, leave them out. You could also substitute your favorite homemade or store-bought dressing; ¼ cup (60 mL) is required to coat the salad. Remember, you do not want it soaked in dressing, just enough to enhance the natural flavors.

Only lavender that has been grown specifically for food use should be used in cooking. Avoid lavender sold for decoration or potpourri, as it may have been treated to preserve the color.

This salad is best served fresh, but it will keep for up to 2 days in the refrigerator.

1 cup	quinoa, well rinsed and drained	250 mL
2 cups	cold water	500 mL
2	tomatoes, chopped	2
2	large sprigs Italian (flat-leaf) parsley (leaves only), chopped	2
¼	English cucumber, chopped	¼
⅓ cup	chopped red, green, yellow or mixed bell peppers	75 mL

Vinaigrette

3 tbsp	extra virgin olive oil	45 mL
2 tbsp	freshly squeezed lemon juice	30 mL
1½ tsp	hot pepper flakes (optional)	7 mL
½ tsp	salt	2 mL
½ tsp	freshly ground black pepper	2 mL
½ tsp	dried lavender flowers (optional)	2 mL

1. In a medium saucepan, over medium heat, bring quinoa and water to a boil. Reduce heat and boil gently for 10 to 15 minutes or until the white germ separates from the seed. Cover, remove from heat and let stand for 5 minutes. Remove lid, let cool and fluff with a fork.

2. Meanwhile, in a large bowl, combine tomatoes, parsley, cucumber and bell peppers. Stir in cooled quinoa.

3. *Vinaigrette:* In a small bowl, whisk together olive oil, lemon juice, hot pepper flakes (if using), salt, pepper and lavender (if using).

4. Pour vinaigrette over salad and toss to coat.

This recipe courtesy of Deloris Del Rio.

Quinoa: Here are a couple more recipe ideas for quinoa:
- Combine chilled cooked quinoa with pinto beans, pumpkin seeds, green onions and cilantro. Season to taste and enjoy this south-of-the-border-inspired salad.
- Add nuts and fruits to cooked quinoa and serve as a breakfast porridge, topped with milk or yogurt.

NUTRIENTS PER SERVING	
Calories	108
Fat	5 g
Carbohydrate	14 g
Fiber	2 g
Protein	3 g

Bulgur Salad with Broccoli, Radishes and Celery

This colorful salad has Middle Eastern flare.

Tip

Cooking the vinegar, mustard and garlic along with the broth intensifies the flavor of the cooked bulgur.

Variations

Use freshly squeezed lemon juice instead of vinegar.

Add ½ cup (125 mL) mixed chopped fresh herbs, such as basil, oregano, tarragon and thyme.

For added protein and fiber, add 1 cup (250 mL) cooked chickpeas, lentils or black beans.

Steamer basket

1½ cups	broccoli florets	375 mL
1	clove garlic, minced	1
¾ cup	reduced-sodium chicken broth	175 mL
3 tbsp	red wine vinegar	45 mL
1½ tsp	Dijon mustard	7 mL
1 cup	bulgur	250 mL
⅓ cup	chopped radishes	75 mL
⅓ cup	chopped celery	75 mL
⅓ cup	chopped red bell pepper	75 mL
¼ cup	chopped green onions	60 mL
1½ tbsp	extra virgin olive oil	22 mL
½ tsp	freshly ground black pepper	2 mL
¼ tsp	salt	1 mL

1. In a large pot fitted with a steamer basket, steam broccoli for 4 to 5 minutes or until tender-crisp. Drain and set aside.

2. In a medium saucepan, combine garlic, broth, vinegar and mustard; bring to a boil over high heat. Remove from heat and stir in bulgur. Cover and let stand for 15 minutes. Fluff with a fork.

3. Add broccoli, radishes, celery, red pepper and green onions to bulgur mixture and stir to combine. Gently stir in oil, pepper and salt.

This recipe courtesy of dietitian Pam Hatton.

Nutrients
PER SERVING

Calories	94
Fat	3 g
Carbohydrate	15 g
Fiber	3 g
Protein	3 g

Vietnamese Chicken and Rice Noodle Salad

Here's a tasty salad that capitalizes on two culinary trends: Vietnamese food and noodles.

Tips

Vietnamese fish sauce (*nuoc nam*) is an integral part of Vietnamese cooking. It is a clear, pungent liquid made by fermenting fish with salt. It takes a little getting used to, but it is a great flavor enhancer in many dishes. Fish sauce is high in sodium, so use it sparingly. Find it and curry paste in the Asian sections of some supermarkets.

Rice noodles are an excellent alternative to pasta for people who do not include gluten in their diets. Serve this tasty salad with fruit-flavored yogurt to increase your intake of calcium.

3½ oz	wide rice noodles (half a 7-oz/210 g package)	105 g
12 oz	shredded cooked chicken	375 g
2 cups	diced cucumbers	500 mL
2 cups	grated carrots	500 mL
1 cup	julienned green bell peppers	250 mL
¼ cup	finely chopped fresh cilantro	60 mL
Dressing		
⅓ cup	fish sauce or sodium-reduced soy sauce	75 mL
¼ cup	rice wine vinegar	60 mL
2 tbsp	lime juice	30 mL
1 to 2 tbsp	curry paste	15 to 30 mL
2 tsp	granulated sugar	10 mL
1 tsp	minced garlic	5 mL
1 tsp	sesame oil	5 mL
½ cup	chopped peanuts (optional)	125 mL

1. In a large pot of boiling water, cook noodles for 5 to 8 minutes or until barely tender; drain. Rinse under cold water; drain. Transfer to a large bowl. Add chicken, cucumbers, carrots, peppers and cilantro.

2. *Dressing:* In a small bowl, blend together fish sauce, vinegar, lime juice, curry paste, sugar, garlic and sesame oil. Add dressing to noodle mixture; toss to combine. Sprinkle with peanuts, if using.

This recipe courtesy of Gaitree Peters.

Nutrients PER SERVING	
Calories	214
Fat	5 g
Carbohydrate	23 g
Fiber	2 g
Protein	19 g

Meat and Poultry Main Dishes

Beef Tenderloin with Blue Cheese Herb Crust

Although it is costly, beef tenderloin is both lean and tender, and there is no waste as there is with some less expensive cuts of meat.

Tips

If fresh thyme is available, use 1 tsp (5 mL) leaves in the sauce instead of the dried thyme.

There are many different types of blue cheese, ranging in flavor from very mild to very strong. You may want to sample some at the cheese counter before deciding which is for you.

In this recipe, the strong tastes of the blue cheese and the garlic complement the lower-fat preparation. Complete this rich-tasting meal with simple and light accompaniments such as parsleyed potatoes and a steamed green vegetable.

- **Preheat oven to 350°F (180°C)**
- **Food processor**
- **Baking sheet**

Sauce

1 cup	beef broth	250 mL
1 tbsp	cornstarch	15 mL
¼ tsp	crushed dried thyme	1 mL

Beef

⅓ cup	crumbled blue cheese	75 mL
¼ cup	fresh white bread crumbs	60 mL
2 tbsp	chopped fresh parsley	30 mL
2 tbsp	chopped fresh chives or green onions	30 mL
1	clove garlic	1
4	beef tenderloin medallions (3 oz/90 g each)	4

1. *Sauce:* In a small saucepan, bring broth, cornstarch and thyme to a boil, stirring; simmer for 1 minute. Keep warm.

2. *Beef:* In food processor, process cheese, crumbs, parsley, chives and garlic until in fine crumbs.

3. In a nonstick skillet, brown medallions quickly on each side. Remove from skillet and place on baking sheet. Pack cheese mixture evenly on top of each. Bake in preheated oven for about 20 minutes for medium doneness or as desired. Spoon sauce onto plates and top with beef.

This recipe courtesy of chef Larry DeVries and dietitians Jackie Kopilas and Rachel Barkley.

Nutrients
PER SERVING

Calories	171
Fat	8 g
Carbohydrate	4 g
Fiber	0 g
Protein	19 g

Beef Stew

This is a hearty classic.

Tips

Potatoes are a good source of soluble fiber.

For added flavor and a source of probiotics, add 1 to 2 lbs (0.5 to 1 kg) of pearl onions.

If you prefer, leave out the potatoes and serve the stew over a bed of rice or on its own with fresh bread on the side to soak up the sauce.

For larger appetites, increase the amount of beef in the recipe to 3 lbs (1.5 kg) and serve with a crusty bun on the side.

2 lbs	stewing beef, cubed	1 kg
1	can (28 oz/796 mL) reduced-sodium diced tomatoes, with juice	1
5	whole cloves	5
3	bay leaves	3
2	3-inch (7.5 cm) cinnamon sticks	2
5 to 6	cloves garlic, peeled	5 to 6
1 tbsp	olive oil	15 mL
	Salt and freshly ground black pepper	
3	large potatoes, peeled and quartered	3

1. In a large, heavy-bottomed pot, combine beef, tomatoes and juice, cloves, bay leaves, cinnamon sticks, garlic, oil and salt and pepper to taste. Add enough water to just cover ingredients. Cover and bring to a boil over high heat. Reduce heat to medium and simmer for 1 hour. Add more water to cover ingredients if necessary.

2. Add potatoes and simmer for 1 hour or until beef and potatoes are tender, most of the liquid has evaporated and mixture has thickened. Remove and discard bay leaves.

Nutrients	
PER SERVING	
Calories	174
Fat	8 g
Carbohydrate	7 g
Fiber	1 g
Protein	18 g

Sunny Day Shepherd's Pie

Makes 6 servings

Shepherd's pie is comfort food at its finest. Traditionally, it was eaten to use up leftover cooked lamb or mutton, gravy and vegetables. Here, it's updated with a sweet potato topping.

Tips

Sweet potatoes are a source of soluble fiber.

Have all your vegetables chopped before you start to cook this recipe.

Variation

Use leftover mashed white potatoes instead of sweet potatoes.

- **Preheat oven to 350°F (180°C)**
- **8-inch (20 cm) square glass baking dish**

1 lb	extra-lean ground beef	500 g
1/2 cup	chopped onion	125 mL
1/2 cup	chopped carrot	125 mL
1/2 cup	chopped celery	125 mL
1/2 tsp	freshly ground black pepper	2 mL
1/4 tsp	salt	1 mL
1/4 tsp	ground nutmeg	1 mL
1	clove garlic, minced	1
1 1/2 tbsp	all-purpose flour	22 mL
1 1/4 cups	reduced-sodium beef broth	300 mL
1/2 cup	drained no-salt-added canned corn	125 mL
2 cups	mashed sweet potatoes (about 2 medium)	500 mL

1. In a large skillet, over medium-high heat, cook beef, breaking it up with the back of a spoon, for about 8 minutes or until no longer pink. Using a slotted spoon, transfer beef to a bowl and set aside. Drain off all but 2 tsp (10 mL) fat from the pan.

2. Reduce heat to medium. Add onion, carrot, celery, pepper, salt and nutmeg to the skillet and sauté for 4 to 5 minutes or until vegetables are softened. Add garlic and sauté for 30 seconds. Sprinkle with flour and cook, stirring, for 1 minute. Gradually stir in broth and bring to a boil; boil, stirring, until thickened. Return beef and accumulated juices to the pan and stir to coat.

3. Pour beef mixture into baking dish. Sprinkle corn evenly over top. Spread sweet potatoes evenly over corn.

4. Bake in preheated oven for 35 to 40 minutes or until a knife inserted in the center comes out hot.

This recipe courtesy of Jennifer Lactin.

Nutrients
PER SERVING

Calories	241
Fat	7 g
Carbohydrate	26 g
Fiber	4 g
Protein	19 g

Braised Roasted Veal

This marvelously moist dish (which you can make the day before) is excellent served as part of a cold buffet with salads and bread.

Tips

If making this dish ahead of time, refrigerate the veal in a clean container within 2 hours of cooking.

Using vegetables, herbs and lemon to flavor the meat in this recipe increases the taste without increasing the fat content.

- **Preheat oven to 475°F (240°C)**
- **Roasting pan**

2 lb	veal leg (top portion)	1 kg
½ tsp	crumbled dried rosemary	2 mL
½ tsp	dried thyme	2 mL
Pinch	dried tarragon	Pinch
1	stalk celery, chopped	1
1	onion, chopped	1
1	carrot, diced	1
⅓ cup	water	75 mL
¼ cup	white vinegar	60 mL
¼ cup	white wine	60 mL
1 tsp	grated lemon zest	5 mL
1 tbsp	freshly squeezed lemon juice	15 mL

1. Place veal in roasting pan; sprinkle with rosemary, thyme and tarragon. Place celery, onion and carrot around veal. Roast in preheated oven for 10 minutes.

2. Reduce temperature to 375°F (190°C). Add water, vinegar, wine, lemon zest and juice. Cover and roast for 1 hour. Remove from pan and cool. Chill. Slice to serve.

This recipe courtesy of chef Ronald Davis and dietitian Debra McNair.

Nutrients
PER SERVING

Calories	144
Fat	4 g
Carbohydrate	0 g
Fiber	0 g
Protein	25 g

Mustard Lamb Chops

These succulent chops roast in 10 to 15 minutes, so this recipe is great when you're short on time.

Tip

Serve on a bed of steamed rice or with mashed or oven-roasted potatoes. Add vegetables to complete the meal.

- **Preheat oven to 500°F (260°C)**
- **Shallow roasting pan, lightly greased**

8	lamb loin chops (1 inch/2.5 cm thick), trimmed	8
	Freshly ground black pepper	
⅓ cup	grainy mustard	75 mL

1. Season lamb chops all over with pepper. Arrange in a single layer in prepared roasting pan. Spread about half the mustard over tops of lamb chops. Let stand for 10 to 15 minutes.

2. Bake in preheated oven for 5 minutes or until browned. Turn chops and spread remaining mustard over tops. Bake for 5 minutes for medium-rare or to desired doneness.

Nutrients PER SERVING	
Calories	224
Fat	8 g
Carbohydrate	2 g
Fiber	0 g
Protein	32 g

Pork Tenderloin

Makes 8 servings

This dish is great for company and family dinners.

Tip

Serve with oven-roasted potatoes, steamed rice or quinoa and vegetables.

- **Preheat oven to 450°F (230°C)**
- **Large, heavy-bottomed ovenproof skillet**

2 lbs	pork tenderloin, trimmed	1 kg
	Salt and freshly ground black pepper	
1/3 cup	olive oil, divided	75 mL
1 1/3 cups	canned whole-berry cranberry sauce	325 mL
1 cup	chicken broth	250 mL
1/4 cup	balsamic vinegar	60 mL
2 tbsp	chopped fresh rosemary	30 mL

1. Sprinkle pork all over with salt and pepper. In skillet, heat 1/4 cup (60 mL) of the oil over medium-high heat. Sear pork for 2 minutes on each side. Transfer skillet to preheated oven and bake, uncovered, for 35 minutes or until a meat thermometer inserted in the thickest part of the tenderloin registers 160°F (71°C).

2. Meanwhile, in a small saucepan, heat remaining oil over medium-high heat. Whisk in cranberry sauce, broth, vinegar and rosemary for about 2 minutes or until cranberry sauce has melted. Reduce heat to low and keep warm.

3. Transfer pork to a cutting board. Cover with foil and let rest for 10 minutes.

4. Pour cooking juices and any scrapings from skillet into cranberry mixture and bring to a boil over medium heat. Cook, stirring occasionally, for 15 to 20 minutes or until thickened enough to generously coat a spoon. Season to taste with salt and pepper.

5. Slice pork and serve with sauce.

Nutrients
PER SERVING

Calories	251
Fat	7 g
Carbohydrate	20 g
Fiber	1 g
Protein	26 g

Sweet-and-Sour Pork

This combination of sweet and sour flavors is often featured in Asian dishes.

Tips

Trim as much fat and silverskin as you can from the pork.

When browning the pork, be sure it lifts easily before you turn it, to avoid sticking.

A Dutch oven is a large, heavy pot with a tight-fitting lid. It is most often used to prepare stews. Here, it works well to brown the meat and provides ample room for the added ingredients.

Variation

For a leaner version, use medallions of pork tenderloin instead of pork shoulder; reduce the simmering time to 10 minutes.

Nutrients
PER SERVING

Calories	244
Fat	8 g
Carbohydrate	23 g
Fiber	1 g
Protein	21 g

- **Dutch oven**

3 tbsp	all-purpose flour	45 mL
½ tsp	freshly ground black pepper	2 mL
2 lbs	boneless pork shoulder, trimmed of fat and cut into 1-inch (2.5 cm) pieces	1 kg
2 tbsp	canola oil, divided	30 mL
2	cloves garlic, minced	2
2 cups	diced celery	500 mL
2 cups	reduced-sodium chicken broth, divided	500 mL
1	can (14 oz/398 mL) pineapple chunks, with juice	1
1	red bell pepper, cut into thin strips	1
3 tbsp	cornstarch	45 mL
¼ cup	granulated sugar	60 mL
½ cup	white vinegar	125 mL
1 tbsp	reduced-sodium soy sauce	15 mL

1. In a large, shallow bowl, combine flour and pepper. Dredge pork in seasoned flour, shaking off excess, and place on a clean plate. Discard any excess flour mixture.

2. In a Dutch oven, heat 1 tbsp (15 mL) oil over medium-high heat. Add half the pork and cook for 3 to 4 minutes or until well browned on all sides. Transfer pork to a clean plate. Repeat with the remaining oil and pork.

3. Return all pork and accumulated juices to pot. Add garlic and celery; sauté for 1 minute. Pour in 1 cup (250 mL) of the broth and deglaze the pot, scraping up any browned bits. Stir in pineapple with juice and bring to a boil. Reduce heat to low, cover with a tight-fitting lid and simmer, stirring occasionally, for 20 minutes. Stir in red pepper, cover and simmer for 10 minutes or until pork is tender.

4. Meanwhile, in a medium bowl, whisk cornstarch into the remaining broth. Whisk in sugar, vinegar and soy sauce, whisking until sugar is dissolved. Stir into pot and simmer, stirring, for about 5 minutes or until sauce is thick.

This recipe courtesy of dietitian Anne Taylor.

Yogurt-Marinated Chicken

Makes 8 servings

Here's an interesting variation on tandoori chicken, an Indian specialty. Serve with rice pilaf and a green salad.

Tips

Instead of using chicken breasts only, you can substitute one 3-lb (1.5 kg) chicken, cut into 8 pieces; bake for 45 to 60 minutes.

Most marinated recipes call for vinegar, lemon juice or wine. This Indian-style recipe uses yogurt, which enhances the taste and tenderizes the texture.

- **Preheat oven to 350°F (180°C)**
- **Large metal baking pan**

1¼ cups	low-fat plain yogurt	300 mL
3	cloves garlic, minced	3
1 tbsp	minced gingerroot (or 2 tsp/10 mL ground ginger)	15 mL
1 tbsp	freshly squeezed lemon juice	15 mL
1 tbsp	vegetable oil	15 mL
2 tsp	paprika	10 mL
1 tsp	chili powder	5 mL
1 tsp	crumbled dried rosemary	5 mL
1 tsp	freshly ground black pepper	5 mL
½ tsp	ground turmeric	2 mL
8	boneless skinless chicken breasts (about 1½ lbs/750 g)	8

1. In a large bowl, combine yogurt, garlic, ginger, lemon juice, oil, paprika, chili powder, rosemary, pepper and turmeric; whisk until smooth. Add chicken, turning to coat all over. Cover and refrigerate for 24 hours.

2. Place chicken in single layer in baking pan, reserving marinade. Bake in preheated oven for 20 to 25 minutes or until no longer pink inside, spooning additional marinade over chicken halfway through baking.

This recipe courtesy of chef Nanak Chand Vig and dietitian Fabiola Masri.

Nutrients
PER SERVING

Calories	129
Fat	3 g
Carbohydrate	3 g
Fiber	0 g
Protein	21 g

Brined and Tender Lemon Roast Chicken

Makes 6 servings

Add this tender lean meat as part of your balanced meal.

Tips

If you present the dinner plates with the chicken already portioned, everyone eats less and the remaining chicken can be served at another meal.

Brining chicken in a mild salt solution produces delightfully tender meat. Do not brine the chicken for longer than 8 hours. Over-brining may adversely affect the texture of the cooked chicken.

Tenting the chicken with foil and letting it rest before carving allows the juices to redistribute throughout the meat, creating a much moister chicken.

- **Roasting pan**

1	whole roasting chicken (3 to 4 lbs/1.5 to 2 kg)	1
3 tbsp	kosher salt	45 mL
12 cups	water	3 L
1	lemon	1
2 tsp	canola or olive oil	10 mL
$\frac{1}{2}$ tsp	salt	2 mL

1. Trim excess fat from chicken. Rinse inside and out under cold running water.

2. In a large pot, combine kosher salt and water, stirring to dissolve salt. Add chicken, breast side down, making sure it is fully submerged. Cover and refrigerate for at least 4 hours or for up to 8 hours.

3. About 30 minutes before cooking, drain brine from chicken and discard. Rinse chicken under running water and pat dry. Place on a clean plate and let stand at room temperature.

4. Place oven rack in center of oven, place empty roasting pan on rack and preheat oven to 425°F (220°C).

5. Meanwhile, place whole lemon in a small saucepan and add water to cover. Bring to a boil over high heat. Reduce heat and simmer for 5 minutes. Remove from heat and leave lemon in hot water until ready to use.

6. Rub chicken all over with oil and sprinkle with $\frac{1}{2}$ tsp (2 mL) salt. Remove the lemon from the hot water, discarding water. Poke several holes in the lemon and insert it into the cavity of the chicken.

Nutrients
PER SERVING

Calories	168
Fat	8 g
Carbohydrate	1 g
Fiber	0 g
Protein	23 g

Place a baking dish of pierced, scrubbed small sweet potatoes in the oven next to the roasting pan during the final hour of cooking the chicken. Simply add a salad and dinner is done!

Variation

For added flavor, insert fresh or dried herbs, such as thyme, rosemary, savory or marjoram, into the cavity of the chicken along with the lemon.

7. Carefully remove the hot roasting pan from the oven, place chicken, breast side up, in pan, and roast for 30 minutes. Reduce heat to 400°F (200°C). Roast chicken for 60 minutes or until skin is dark golden and crispy, drumsticks wiggle when touched and a meat thermometer inserted in the thickest part of a thigh registers 165°F (74°C). Transfer chicken to a cutting board, tent with foil and let rest for 10 to 15 minutes before carving and removing the skin.

8. Using kitchen tongs, remove lemon from the chicken. Cut lemon in half and squeeze juice over hot chicken pieces.

This recipe courtesy of dietitian Joanne Rankin.

> **Brining:** Brining is an effective way to add flavor and moisture to meats. The light salt solution helps to loosen the meat muscle fibers, making them more tender. The salt also helps the meat retain some water from the brine, again helping to tenderize. Any flavors in the brine will also infuse into the meat, adding flavor to the final product. With the focus on reducing sodium intake, eat brined meats only occasionally and accompany them with lower-sodium options.

Chicken Florentine

Spinach gives this Italian chicken dish a punch of antioxidants.

Tips

Serve with gluten-free pasta or rice and a second vegetable to complete this meal.

To make ahead: Follow steps 1 through 8, then cover and refrigerate. Remove from refrigerator and let sit at room temperature for 15 minutes before broiling.

- **13- by 9-inch (33 by 23 cm) baking dish**

4 tsp	garlic-infused olive oil, divided	20 mL
1	package (11 oz/312 g) fresh baby spinach	1
1½ lbs	boneless skinless chicken breasts	750 g
	Salt and freshly ground black pepper	
1 tbsp	cornstarch	15 mL
1 tbsp	cold water	15 mL
2 cups	chicken broth	500 mL
1½ cups	water	375 mL
2 tbsp	1% or 2% milk	30 mL
1 tbsp	freshly squeezed lemon juice	15 mL
1 tsp	lemon extract	5 mL
⅓ cup	grated low-fat Parmesan cheese	75 mL

1. In a large skillet, heat 2 tsp (10 mL) of the oil over medium heat. One handful at a time, add spinach and cook until wilted. Transfer to a colander. Let stand until cool enough to handle. Using palms, press out excess water.

2. Season chicken breasts all over with salt and pepper.

3. Wipe skillet clean with paper towels. Heat remaining oil over medium-high heat. Brown chicken, turning once halfway through, for 4 to 6 minutes or until browned all over. Transfer to a plate, cover with foil and keep warm.

4. In a small bowl, stir together cornstarch and 1 tbsp (15 mL) cold water until cornstarch has dissolved.

5. In skillet, whisk together broth, 1½ cups (375 mL) water and cornstarch mixture.

6. Return chicken and juices to skillet and bring to a simmer over medium-high heat. Reduce heat to medium-low, cover and cook, turning once halfway through, for 10 to 15 minutes or until no longer pink in center of thickest part. Using tongs, transfer chicken to a plate and tent loosely with foil.

Nutrients
PER SERVING

Calories	159
Fat	4 g
Carbohydrate	6 g
Fiber	2 g
Protein	25 g

Tip

Choose skinless chicken breasts. Chicken skins add unnecessary fat.

7. Increase heat to medium-high and cook sauce for 15 minutes or until thickened and reduced to about $\frac{3}{4}$ cup (175 mL). Remove from heat. Whisk in milk, lemon juice and lemon extract. Season to taste with salt and pepper.

8. Cut chicken into $\frac{1}{2}$-inch (1 cm) slices and arrange in a single layer in ovenproof baking dish. Spread spinach evenly over chicken and pour sauce over spinach. Sprinkle evenly with cheese.

9. Place an oven rack just below element and turn broiler on high.

10. Broil for about 5 minutes or until cheese is golden brown.

Chicken in Butter Sauce

Indian butter chicken is a favorite the world over. The traditional recipe is very high in fat, with lots of butter and whipping cream. We have reduced the fat content without losing any of the flavor. The ingredient list looks long, but the recipe is really quite simple and is worth the effort.

Tips

Tandoori paste is available in the ethnic food aisle of most supermarkets.

Use the side of a spoon to scrape off the skin of gingerroot before chopping or grating. Gingerroot keeps well in the freezer for up to 3 months and can be grated from frozen.

Serve over steamed basmati rice, garnished with chopped fresh cilantro. Accompany with steamed green beans or asparagus.

Nutrients
PER SERVING

Calories	175
Fat	6 g
Carbohydrate	5 g
Fiber	1 g
Protein	24 g

- **11- by 7-inch (28 by 18 cm) baking pan**

3 tbsp	tandoori paste (see tip, at left)	45 mL
2 tbsp	freshly squeezed lemon juice	30 mL
2 tbsp	low-fat plain yogurt	30 mL
1½ lbs	boneless skinless chicken breasts, cut into 1-inch (2.5 cm) chunks	750 g

Sauce

¼ cup	tomato paste	60 mL
½ cup	water	125 mL
1	1-inch (2.5 cm) cube gingerroot, very finely grated	1
1	fresh green chile pepper, seeded and finely chopped	1
4 tsp	freshly squeezed lemon juice	20 mL
1 tbsp	chopped fresh cilantro	15 mL
1 tsp	ground cumin	5 mL
1 tsp	garam masala	5 mL
¾ tsp	salt	3 mL
¼ tsp	granulated sugar	1 mL
¼ tsp	chili powder	1 mL
1 tbsp	unsalted butter	15 mL
1 cup	half-and-half (10%) cream	250 mL

1. In a large bowl, combine tandoori paste, lemon juice and yogurt. Add chicken and stir well to coat. Cover and refrigerate for at least 1 hour or overnight. Preheat oven to 350°F (180°C).

2. Arrange chicken in a single layer in baking pan and pour in marinade. Bake for 20 to 25 minutes or until no longer pink inside.

3. *Sauce:* Meanwhile, in a small bowl, combine tomato paste and water. Stir in ginger, chile pepper, lemon juice, cilantro, cumin, garam masala, salt, sugar and chili powder.

4. In a large saucepan, melt butter over medium heat. Stir in sauce and bring to a simmer. Add cooked chicken and any juice from the baking pan; simmer for about 10 minutes to combine flavors. Add cream and cook for 3 minutes to heat through (do not boil).

This recipe courtesy of Eileen Campbell.

Chicken Vegetable Lasagna

Lasagna is always a popular dish for parties and buffets, and this version, which features chicken and a variety of vegetables instead of ground beef, is both light and satisfying.

Tips

If desired, substitute lean ground turkey for the chicken.

This is a lower-fat, higher-fiber alternative to traditional lasagna. Chicken, rather than ground beef, provides the protein. Replacing the traditional white sauce or ricotta cheese with vegetables lowers the fat and adds fiber and vitamins.

Nutrients	
PER SERVING	
Calories	348
Fat	9 g
Carbohydrate	48 g
Fiber	5 g
Protein	21 g

- **Preheat oven to 350°F (180°C)**
- **13- by 9-inch (33 by 23 cm) baking dish**

8 oz	lean ground chicken	250 g
½ cup	chopped onion	125 mL
2	cloves garlic, minced	2
1 tbsp	vegetable oil	15 mL
1 tsp	margarine	5 mL
1	can (28 oz/796 mL) tomatoes	1
1	can (5½ oz/156 mL) tomato paste	1
¾ cup	water	175 mL
1½ tsp	salt	7 mL
Pinch	freshly ground black pepper	Pinch
4	carrots, diced	4
1	bunch broccoli, chopped	1
8 oz	mushrooms, sliced	250 g
¼ cup	chopped fresh parsley	60 mL
12 oz	lasagna noodles	375 g
1	package (6 oz/175 g) sliced part-skim mozzarella cheese	1
	Freshly grated Parmesan cheese	

1. In a saucepan over medium-high heat, cook chicken, onion and garlic in oil and margarine until chicken is no longer pink. Add tomatoes, tomato paste, water, salt and pepper. Cook, uncovered, over medium heat for about 15 minutes, stirring occasionally. Add carrots, broccoli, mushrooms and parsley. Cook, covered, over low heat for about 30 minutes or until mixture is thickened.

2. In a large pot of boiling water, cook noodles according to package directions or until tender but firm; drain well.

3. Spoon one-quarter of the sauce into baking dish. Place one-third of the lasagna noodles over sauce. Repeat layers twice, ending with sauce. Top with cheese slices; sprinkle lightly with Parmesan cheese. Bake in preheated oven for about 30 minutes. Let stand for 10 minutes before serving.

This recipe courtesy of Lisa Raitano.

Pad Thai

Thailand's national dish is just as popular in North America.

Tips

For ¾ cup (175 mL) lime juice, you'll need 6 to 8 limes.

Keep a detailed food diary to accurately assess the types and quantity of food you consume on a daily basis. You can then tailor your diet after analyzing your diary.

- **Blender or food processor**

1¼ cups	chopped fresh cilantro, divided	300 mL
2 tbsp	soy sauce, divided	30 mL
¾ cup	freshly squeezed lime juice, divided	175 mL
1 tbsp	freshly ground black pepper	15 mL
6	boneless skinless chicken breasts (each 4 to 5 oz/125 to 150 g)	6
1 tbsp	garlic-infused olive oil or unflavored olive oil	15 mL
7 oz	broad rice vermicelli noodles	210 g
½ cup	tomato sauce	125 mL
¼ cup	packed brown sugar	60 mL
1 tsp	hot chili sauce	5 mL
2	eggs, lightly beaten	2
2 cups	bean sprouts	500 mL
2 tbsp	finely chopped roasted peanuts	30 mL
2	green onions, thinly sliced	2

1. In blender, blend 1 cup (250 mL) of the cilantro, 1 tbsp (15 mL) of the soy sauce, ¼ cup (60 mL) of the lime juice and pepper until smooth. Pour into a shallow dish. Place chicken in cilantro mixture, turning to coat. Cover and refrigerate for at least 2 hours or overnight.

2. Discarding marinade, remove chicken and slice into 1-inch (2.5 cm) strips. In a large skillet, heat oil and stir-fry chicken strips for 6 to 8 minutes or until no longer pink inside. Transfer to a plate. Set aside and keep warm.

3. In a large pot of boiling water, cook vermicelli according to package instructions. Drain and set aside.

4. In a small bowl, stir together tomato sauce, brown sugar, chili sauce, remaining soy sauce and remaining lime juice.

5. Transfer tomato sauce mixture to a large skillet and bring to a simmer. Add eggs and let set slightly before stirring into sauce. Gently toss in noodles until coated. Gently toss in chicken and bean sprouts.

6. Transfer to a serving platter. Garnish with peanuts, green onions and remaining cilantro.

Nutrients
PER SERVING

Calories	300
Fat	7 g
Carbohydrate	32 g
Fiber	2 g
Protein	29 g

Thai Turkey Stir-Fry

This recipe is a great introduction to Thai cuisine. It's not too spicy, so it appeals to all ages.

Tip

Serve over jasmine rice or whole wheat pasta. Finish the meal with tropical fruits, such as mango, pineapple and papaya.

1 tbsp	vegetable oil	15 mL
2	cloves garlic, finely chopped	2
1	2-inch (5 cm) piece gingerroot, grated	1
1 lb	boneless skinless turkey breast, cut into strips	500 g
1	head bok choy (about 1 lb/500 g), chopped	1
1	red bell pepper, julienned	1
½ cup	light coconut milk	125 mL
1 tsp	grated lime zest	5 mL
2 tbsp	freshly squeezed lime juice	30 mL
1 tbsp	reduced-sodium soy sauce	15 mL
1 tsp	red curry paste	5 mL
	Salt and freshly ground black pepper	
2 tsp	chopped fresh cilantro	10 mL

1. Heat a wok or large skillet over medium-high heat. Add oil and swirl to coat wok. Sauté garlic, ginger and turkey for about 10 minutes or until turkey is lightly browned on the outside and no longer pink inside. Add bok choy and red pepper; sauté for 4 minutes. Stir in coconut milk, lime zest, lime juice, soy sauce and curry paste; bring to a boil. Reduce heat and simmer for 10 minutes or until sauce has thickened slightly. Season to taste with salt and pepper.

2. Ladle onto plates and garnish with cilantro.

This recipe courtesy of Amélie Roy-Fleming and Marie-Eve Richard.

Nutrients
PER SERVING

Calories	227
Fat	8 g
Carbohydrate	10 g
Fiber	3 g
Protein	30 g

Spicy Brown Rice Jambalaya

Makes 8 servings

Jambalaya is a dish native to New Orleans, developed from the traditional Spanish dish paella.

Tips

Themed dinners are a great way to explore new cuisines. Consider making this jambalaya the centerpiece of a Cajun-themed dinner.

Much of the sodium in this recipe comes from the sausages and the canned beans. If you want to reduce the sodium, look for reduced-sodium sausages and use cooked rehydrated dried kidney beans.

Variation

Jambalaya was designed to use up leftovers, so instead of cooking fresh sausage, you could add cooked sausage or chicken to the rice mixture.

2 tsp	canola oil	10 mL
1 lb	lean hot turkey sausages, cut into 1-inch (2.5 cm) pieces	500 g
1	jalapeño pepper, seeded and finely chopped	1
1 cup	chopped red onion	250 mL
1 cup	chopped green bell pepper	250 mL
1 cup	chopped red bell pepper	250 mL
1 cup	chopped celery	250 mL
4	cloves garlic, minced	4
2	bay leaves	2
1 tbsp	Cajun seasoning	15 mL
1 tsp	dried oregano	5 mL
2 tbsp	tomato paste	30 mL
1	can (19 oz/540 mL) kidney beans, drained and rinsed	1
1	can (14 oz/398 mL) diced tomatoes, with juice	1
1½ cups	long-grain brown rice	375 mL
½ cup	coarsely chopped fresh parsley	125 mL

1. In a large, heavy pot, heat oil over medium heat. Sauté sausage for 4 to 5 minutes or until browned on all sides. Transfer to a plate and set aside.

2. Drain off and discard all but 2 tsp (10 mL) fat from pot. Add jalapeño, red onion, green pepper, red pepper and celery; sauté for 5 to 7 minutes or until softened. Add garlic and sauté for 30 seconds. Add bay leaves, Cajun seasoning, oregano and tomato paste; cook, stirring, for 2 minutes.

3. Return sausage to the pot and stir in beans, tomatoes, rice and 3½ cups (875 mL) water; bring to a boil. Reduce heat and simmer, stirring occasionally, for 1¼ hours or until liquid is absorbed and rice is tender. Add more water if rice is chewy. Serve garnished with parsley.

This recipe courtesy of dietitian Giovanna Pizzin.

Nutrients PER SERVING	
Calories	315
Fat	7 g
Carbohydrate	45 g
Fiber	8 g
Protein	18 g

Fish and Seafood Main Dishes

Tasty Fish Cakes

This is a great way to use up leftover cooked salmon and mashed potatoes, but it's just as good made with canned salmon.

Tip

Use plain puréed or mashed potato, without milk or butter added.

Variation

Vary the flavor by using 6 oz (175 g) cooked haddock, crab or diced shrimp instead of salmon. Change the herbs and veggies depending on the fish or seafood you choose.

1	can (7½ oz/213 g) salmon, drained, skin and large bones removed (or 6 oz/175 g leftover cooked salmon)	1
1 cup	puréed or mashed potatoes	250 mL
¼ cup	finely chopped green onion	60 mL
¼ cup	finely chopped red bell pepper	60 mL
3 tbsp	chopped fresh dill	45 mL
3 tbsp	milk	45 mL
	Salt and freshly ground black pepper	
1	egg, beaten	1
	Vegetable cooking spray	

1. In a medium bowl, combine salmon, potatoes, green onion, red pepper, dill and milk. Season to taste with salt and pepper. Gently stir in egg. Form mixture into four ¾-inch (2 cm) thick cakes. Cover and refrigerate for at least 30 minutes or overnight to let flavor develop.

2. Heat a large nonstick skillet over medium heat. Spray with vegetable cooking spray. Add fish cakes and cook for about 2 minutes per side, or until browned on both sides and hot in the center.

This recipe courtesy of Eileen Campbell.

Nutrients PER SERVING	
Calories	149
Fat	5 g
Carbohydrate	12 g
Fiber	1 g
Protein	13 g

Oven-Baked Fish and Chips

Makes 6 servings

This is a healthier and lighter version of the original deep-fried fish and chips.

Tip

To increase the fiber content, leave the potato skins on. Just be sure to scrub them clean!

- **Preheat oven to 450°F (230°C)**
- **Two rimmed baking sheets, lined with foil**

Oven-Baked Chips

3 lbs	baking potatoes, peeled	1.5 kg
1 tbsp	vegetable oil	15 mL
	Salt and freshly ground black pepper	
2 tsp	dried oregano	10 mL

Oven-Baked Fish

¾ cup	dry bread crumbs	175 mL
2 tsp	dried basil	10 mL
2 tsp	dried oregano	10 mL
	Salt and freshly ground black pepper	
2	eggs, beaten	2
6	skinless cod fillets	6
2 tbsp	vegetable oil	30 mL

1. *Oven-Baked Chips:* In a medium bowl, whisk together oil, salt and pepper to taste and oregano. Cut potatoes into thick fries. Pat dry with paper towels. Toss with oil mixture to coat. Arrange in single layer on a prepared baking sheet.

2. Bake in preheated oven, gently stirring and turning once halfway through, for 40 minutes or until crisp.

3. *Oven-Baked Fish:* In a shallow dish, combine bread crumbs, basil, oregano and salt and pepper to taste. Set aside. Into another shallow dish, pour eggs.

4. Cut fish into 6 same-size pieces. Pat dry with paper towels. One at a time, dip each piece into eggs to coat all over, then dredge in bread crumb mixture to coat all over and transfer to the other prepared baking sheet. Drizzle with oil.

5. Bake in top half of preheated oven, turning once halfway through, for 10 to 14 minutes or until fish is opaque and flakes easily when tested with a fork.

NUTRIENTS PER SERVING

Calories	393
Fat	11 g
Carbohydrate	47 g
Fiber	4 g
Protein	26 g

Fish Roll-Ups

In combination with onions and mushrooms, spinach makes a tasty filling for fish.

Tips

If you prefer, use frozen chopped spinach to replace fresh in this recipe. Just thaw 1 package (10 oz/ 300 g), drain well and squeeze dry. Use half in this recipe and save the remainder for another use.

This recipe is a real winner in the lower-fat category. Complement the delicate blend of sole, spinach and mushrooms with a rice dish and baby carrots to add color and vitamin A.

- **Preheat oven to 425°F (220°C)**
- **Baking pan, lightly greased**

½	package (10 oz/300 g) fresh spinach	½
1	small onion, chopped	1
1 tbsp	margarine	15 mL
1 cup	chopped mushrooms	250 mL
¼ cup	whole wheat bread crumbs	60 mL
1 lb	skinless sole fillets	500 g
	Salt, freshly ground black pepper and dried thyme	
½	lemon	½
	Paprika	

1. Steam spinach until tender; drain well. In a small skillet over medium-high heat, cook onion in margarine for about 5 minutes or until browned. Add mushrooms; cook for 3 minutes. In a food processor, combine spinach, mushroom mixture and bread crumbs. Process using on/ off motion until coarsely chopped.

2. Season fish fillets with salt, pepper and thyme to taste. (If fish fillets are too wide, cut in half down center.) Spoon spinach filling over each fillet; roll up and secure with toothpicks. Place fish seam side down in prepared baking pan. Squeeze lemon over fish; sprinkle with paprika. Bake, uncovered, in preheated oven for 10 minutes per inch (2.5 cm) of thickness or until fish flakes easily with fork. Remove toothpicks and serve.

This recipe courtesy of Pamela Najman.

Nutrients
PER SERVING

Calories	144
Fat	4 g
Carbohydrate	8 g
Fiber	1 g
Protein	19 g

Tandoori Haddock

Purchased tandoori paste makes an easy marinade for white fish. This Indian-inspired dish can be made quickly for a great weeknight meal.

Tips

Most supermarkets now carry tandoori paste. You can usually find it in the ethnic food aisle where Indian and Asian sauces are displayed.

For a balanced meal, serve with basmati rice and steamed sugar snap peas.

Variation

This works well with most firm white fish fillets or steaks, such as halibut or orange roughy. It's even great with salmon! Adjust the broiling time depending on the thickness of the fish.

- **Rimmed baking sheet, lightly greased**

¼ cup	tandoori paste (see tip, at left)	60 mL
¼ cup	low-fat yogurt	60 mL
1 tbsp	freshly squeezed lemon juice	15 mL
4	haddock fillets (about 14 oz/420 g total)	4

1. In a shallow dish, combine tandoori paste, yogurt and lemon juice. Add fish, turning to coat evenly. Cover and refrigerate for 20 to 30 minutes. Meanwhile, preheat broiler, with rack set 4 inches (10 cm) from the top.

2. Place fish on baking sheet and broil for 10 minutes or until fish is opaque and flakes easily with a fork and the top is lightly browned.

This recipe courtesy of Eileen Campbell.

Nutrients
PER SERVING

Calories	113
Fat	1 g
Carbohydrate	4 g
Fiber	0 g
Protein	20 g

Teriyaki Halibut

This is an ultra-low-fat fish for special occasions.

Tips

Serve with noodles, oven-roasted potatoes or steamed rice. Add vegetables to round out the meal.

For 6 tbsp (90 mL) lime juice, you'll need 3 to 6 limes.

Protein will keep you feeling full. Choose lean sources of protein where possible.

- **Preheat oven to 400°F (200°C)**
- **Rimmed baking sheet, lined with foil**

	Juice of 2 limes	
2 tbsp	teriyaki sauce	30 mL
2 tsp	olive oil	10 mL
¼ tsp	freshly ground black pepper	1 mL
¼ tsp	paprika	1 mL
1 tsp	fennel seeds, crushed	5 mL
4	skinless halibut fillets	4

1. In a small bowl, whisk together lime juice, teriyaki sauce, oil, pepper, paprika and fennel seeds.

2. In a shallow dish, arrange fillets in single layer. Pour lime juice mixture over fillets, turning to coat. Cover, refrigerate and let marinate for 1 hour.

3. Arrange fillets in single layer on prepared baking sheet. Bake in preheated oven for 20 minutes or until fish is opaque and flakes easily when tested with a fork.

Nutrients PER SERVING	
Calories	257
Fat	7 g
Carbohydrate	4 g
Fiber	0 g
Protein	42 g

Cedar-Baked Salmon

Cedar shingles and shims, available at lumberyards, impart a unique flavor to salmon when baking. For this recipe, you'll need to soak 2 untreated cedar shingles or 1 package cedar shims in water for at least 2 hours or preferably overnight.

Tips

Wood or wood chips, such as mesquite or grape vines, are often used in barbecuing to add flavor to foods.

Soaking the wood ensures that it is damp enough to produce lots of aromatic smoke. When soaking shingles or shims, weight them down. Otherwise they will float to the surface.

Salmon is a source of omega-3 fatty acids. Accompanied by a rice dish and an array of vegetables, this recipe is a winner.

Nutrients PER SERVING	
Calories	181
Fat	7 g
Carbohydrate	7 g
Fiber	3 g
Protein	23 g

- **Preheat oven to 425°F (220°C)**
- **Soaked cedar shingles or shims**
- **Steamer basket**

1½ lbs	salmon fillets	750 g
	Grated zest and juice of 1 lime	
1½ cups	diagonally sliced asparagus	375 mL
¼ cup	julienned leek	60 mL
4	thin slices red onion	4
¼ cup	diagonally sliced celery	60 mL
½ cup	thickly sliced shiitake mushrooms	125 mL
2	tomatoes, seeded and cut into strips	2
8	fresh basil leaves, slivered	8
1	bag (10 oz/300 g) fresh spinach, trimmed	1
	Salt and freshly ground black pepper	

1. Place soaked shingles or shims on baking sheet; lightly brush with oil. Remove skin and any bones from salmon; cut into 6 serving-size pieces and place on cedar. Sprinkle with lime zest and juice. Bake in preheated oven for 10 to 15 minutes or until fish flakes easily when tested with fork.

2. Meanwhile, in steamer basket, combine asparagus, leek, onion and celery; steam until partially cooked. Add mushrooms, tomatoes, basil and spinach; steam just until tender-crisp and spinach has wilted. Place on 6 individual plates; season with salt and pepper to taste. Top each with salmon.

This recipe courtesy of chef Judson Simpson and dietitian Violaine Sauvé.

Maple Ginger Salmon

This is a North American twist on an Asian classic.

- Preheat oven to 350°F (180°C)
- Rimmed baking sheet, lined with foil

4	skinless salmon fillets	4
¼ cup	pure maple syrup	60 mL
2 tbsp	rice vinegar	30 mL
1 tsp	finely grated gingerroot	5 mL

1. Place salmon on prepared baking sheet.
2. In a small bowl, whisk together maple syrup, vinegar, and ginger. Pour over fillets.
3. Bake in preheated oven for 10 to 15 minutes or until fish is opaque and flakes easily when tested with a fork.

Nutrients
PER SERVING

Calories	319
Fat	12 g
Carbohydrate	14 g
Fiber	0 g
Protein	37 g

Peachy Glazed Trout

The delicate flavor of peaches and their pleasant orange color complement trout beautifully.

Tips

The blanching time of the peaches will vary depending on their ripeness.

Fatty fish, such as trout, salmon, mackerel and herring, are good sources of omega-3 fats.

Variations

Use nectarines or plums, adjusting the blanching time to suit the ripeness of the fruit.

Use salmon or arctic char instead of trout and increase the cooking time as necessary.

- **Preheat oven to 400°F (200°C)**
- **13- by 9-inch (33 by 23 cm) glass baking dish, greased**

3	peaches	3
1	clove garlic, minced	1
2 tsp	grated gingerroot	10 mL
2 tbsp	lightly packed brown sugar	30 mL
½ tsp	freshly ground black pepper	2 mL
⅓ cup	unsweetened orange juice	75 mL
1 tbsp	reduced-sodium soy sauce	15 mL
1 tbsp	Dijon mustard	15 mL
6	skinless trout fillets (about 1½ lbs/750 g total)	6

1. Using a paring knife, make a small X at the bottom of each peach. In a medium saucepan of simmering water, blanch peaches for 2 to 3 minutes or until skins begin to peel back. Using a slotted spoon, transfer peaches to ice water to stop the cooking process. Let cool for 5 minutes or until cool enough to handle. Peel off and discard skin. Chop peaches.

2. In a medium bowl, combine peaches, garlic, ginger, brown sugar, pepper, orange juice, soy sauce and mustard.

3. Pat trout fillets dry with paper towels. Place in prepared baking dish and pour sauce evenly over fish.

4. Bake in preheated oven, basting occasionally with sauce, for 12 to 15 minutes or until fish is opaque and flakes easily when tested with a fork.

This recipe courtesy of Compass Group Canada.

Nutrients
PER SERVING

Calories	203
Fat	6 g
Carbohydrate	11 g
Fiber	1 g
Protein	25 g

Italian Seafood Stew

This is a great dinner party dish that is easy to put together yet tastes like you've been slaving all day over the stove.

Tip

Serve with crusty Italian bread for dunking and have biscotti and a latte for dessert.

Variation

If you cannot find or do not like fennel, substitute 3 stalks celery, thinly sliced, and garnish with the leaves.

½	fennel bulb	½
2 tbsp	olive oil	30 mL
2	cloves garlic, crushed	2
1	large onion, diced	1
1	red bell pepper, diced	1
4 cups	Big-Batch Italian Tomato Master Sauce (page 234) or good-quality commercial marinara sauce	1 L
	Juice of 1 lemon	
1½ lbs	large shrimp, peeled and deveined	750 g
8 oz	mussels, in shell	250 g
1 lb	halibut fillets, skin removed and cut into chunks	500 g
1 tbsp	hot pepper sauce (optional)	15 mL
2 tbsp	chopped fresh parsley	30 mL

1. Remove stalks, base and hard core of fennel, reserving the fronds (feathery leaves). Chop the remainder into 1-inch (2.5 cm) chunks. Chop 2 tbsp (30 mL) of the fronds and set aside.

2. In a large saucepan, heat oil over medium heat. Sauté fennel chunks, garlic, onion and red pepper until onion is lightly browned, about 5 minutes. Add tomato sauce and bring to a boil. Reduce heat, cover and simmer for 5 minutes. Stir in lemon juice. Add shrimp, mussels and halibut; cover and simmer for 5 to 10 minutes or until shrimp are pink and opaque, mussels have opened and halibut is opaque. Discard any mussels that do not open. Add hot pepper sauce, if using.

3. Ladle into bowls and sprinkle with parsley and fennel fronds.

This recipe courtesy of Eileen Campbell.

Nutrients PER SERVING	
Calories	214
Fat	7 g
Carbohydrate	11 g
Fiber	2 g
Protein	26 g

Pasta with White Clam Sauce

Pasta with clams is an Italian classic and for good reason — it's as good to eat as it is easy to make.

Tips

Fresh clams are superb in this dish. Substitute 2 cups (500 mL) fresh shucked clams for the canned clams. Instead of the reserved clam juice, use ¾ cup (175 mL) fish or vegetable stock.

For a change of color, try making this with red clam sauce: just add 1 cup (250 mL) chopped tomatoes to the sauce at the end of step 1.

When recipes call for cream, try replacing it with 2% evaporated milk, which is lower in fat and higher in calcium. Keep some in your pantry so you will always have it on hand.

1 tbsp	olive oil	15 mL
¼ cup	chopped onions	60 mL
2 cups	sliced mushrooms	500 mL
2 tsp	all-purpose flour	10 mL
⅓ cup	dry white wine	75 mL
2	cans (each 5 oz/142 g) clams, drained (reserve ¾ cup/175 mL clam juice)	2
1 tsp	minced garlic	5 mL
1	can (5½ oz/156 mL) 2% evaporated milk	1
⅛ tsp	ground nutmeg	0.5 mL
8 oz	capellini or vermicelli	250 g
2 tbsp	chopped fresh parsley (or 2 tsp/10 mL dried)	30 mL
	Freshly ground black pepper	

1. In a large nonstick skillet, heat oil over medium-high heat. Add onions and mushrooms; sauté for 5 to 6 minutes or until softened and moisture has evaporated. Sprinkle with flour; blend well. Add wine, reserved clam juice and garlic; bring to a boil. Reduce heat and simmer for 2 to 3 minutes or until thickened. Stir in clams, evaporated milk and nutmeg; simmer for 1 to 2 minutes or until heated through.

2. Just before serving, cook pasta according to package directions or until tender but firm; drain. Toss with sauce. Sprinkle with parsley. Season with pepper to taste.

This recipe courtesy of Mary Anne Pucovsky.

Nutrients
PER SERVING

Calories	412
Fat	7 g
Carbohydrate	54 g
Fiber	3 g
Protein	30 g

Scallop Risotto

The delicate flavor of scallops works beautifully with the creamy risotto in this elegant recipe.

Tips

If you use the small bay scallops, they do not need to be cut into smaller pieces. Sea scallops, however, are much larger, up to 2 inches (5 cm) in diameter, and should be cut into smaller pieces for this recipe. Be sure to trim off the tough muscle from the sides of scallops before cutting.

Pancetta, often known as Italian bacon, is high in fat, so use it sparingly.

The scallops are cooked separately so they don't overcook.

Nutrients
PER SERVING

Calories	199
Fat	6 g
Carbohydrate	23 g
Fiber	1 g
Protein	10 g

Risotto

3 cups	reduced-sodium chicken broth	750 mL
1 tsp	olive oil	5 mL
1 tsp	butter	5 mL
1/4 cup	finely diced shallots	60 mL
2	cloves garlic, minced	2
1 cup	Arborio rice	250 mL
1 cup	dry white wine	250 mL
2/3 cup	freshly grated Parmesan cheese	150 mL
Pinch	salt	Pinch
	Freshly ground white pepper	
1 tbsp	chopped fresh thyme (optional)	15 mL

Scallops

2 tsp	olive oil	10 mL
1/4 cup	finely chopped shallots	60 mL
2	cloves garlic, minced	2
1/4 cup	finely diced pancetta	60 mL
1 cup	sea scallops, trimmed and cut into 3/4-inch (2 cm) pieces (see tip, at left)	250 mL

1. *Risotto:* In a saucepan, combine broth and 3 cups (750 mL) water; bring to a simmer over high heat. Reduce heat to low and keep warm.

2. In a medium saucepan, heat oil and butter over medium heat. Sauté shallots for 1 to 2 minutes or until softened but not browned. Add garlic and sauté for 30 seconds. Stir in rice until coated. Add wine and bring to a simmer. Simmer, stirring, until liquid is reduced. Stir in 1 cup (250 mL) broth; simmer, stirring often, until liquid is almost absorbed and the starch from the rice begins to release. Continue to add broth, 1 cup (250 mL) at a time, stirring often, until only 1 cup (250 mL) of broth remains. Make sure broth never completely absorbs into rice between additions.

Tips

If serving this dish as an entrée, simply add some steamed asparagus and carrots to complete the meal.

To serve as an appetizer for 8 people, place risotto in attractive scallop shells that have been transformed into dishes.

Variation

Use small shrimp (size 36 to 45) instead of chopped scallops.

3. *Scallops:* Meanwhile, in a nonstick skillet, heat oil over medium heat. Sauté shallots for 1 to 2 minutes or until softened but not browned. Add garlic and sauté for 30 seconds. Add pancetta and sauté for 5 minutes or until some of the fat is released. Add scallops and sauté for 2 to 3 minutes or until almost firm and opaque. Transfer scallop mixture to a plate and keep warm.

4. Check the consistency of the rice. If al dente, continue to step 5. If not yet al dente, stir in the remaining broth and cook, stirring, until al dente.

5. Stir in scallop mixture, cheese and salt. Season to taste with pepper. Serve garnished with thyme, if using.

This recipe courtesy of Summer-Lee Clark.

> **Rice for Risotto:** Arborio rice is a short-grain rice that is high in starch, making it ideal for risotto. Carnaroli, another short-grain rice, also works well. Rice for risotto should not be rinsed before use, as the starch in the outer coating helps make the risotto creamy.

Stir-Fried Scallops with Curried Sweet Peppers

This is an easy, elegant dish with just a few ingredients. Be careful not to overcook the scallops, as they are delicate.

Tip

This is great served over fine pasta, such as angel hair. Fruit salad and a glass of milk will finish the meal nicely.

2 tbsp	curry powder (or 2 tsp/10 mL mild curry paste)	30 mL
1 tbsp	olive oil, divided	15 mL
Pinch	salt	Pinch
1 lb	sea scallops, halved horizontally	500 g
1	red bell pepper, julienned	1
1	green bell pepper, julienned	1
1	yellow bell pepper, julienned	1
½ cup	white wine, apple juice or water	125 mL
1 tsp	dark sesame oil	5 mL
1 tbsp	chopped fresh cilantro	15 mL

1. In a large bowl, combine curry powder, 1 tsp (5 mL) of the oil and salt. Add scallops and toss to coat.

2. In a wok or a large skillet, heat the remaining oil over medium-high heat. Add scallops and stir-fry for 1 minute. Add red, green and yellow peppers; stir-fry for 1 minute. Add wine and cook, stirring, for 3 to 4 minutes or until scallops are firm and opaque. Stir in sesame oil.

3. Using a slotted spoon, remove scallops and vegetables to a serving bowl. Boil sauce, uncovered, for 3 to 5 minutes, or until thickened. Taste and add salt, if needed.

4. Pour sauce over scallops and vegetables and sprinkle with cilantro. Serve immediately.

This recipe courtesy of dietitian Edie Shaw-Ewald.

Nutrients
PER SERVING

Calories	201
Fat	7 g
Carbohydrate	11 g
Fiber	2 g
Protein	20 g

Easy Shrimp Curry

Makes 2 servings

If you like heat, increase the amount of curry paste in this dish. Serve with brown rice.

Tips

Up to 1 tbsp (15 mL) curry paste can be used, depending on your taste.

When the shrimp is cooked, immediately remove the skillet from the heat to avoid overcooking it.

Fish sauce is a clear brown extraction of salted small fish, such as anchovies, sold in bottles. It is the quintessential ingredient of several Asian cuisines (particularly Thailand's), used to season savory dishes, just as soy sauce is used in Chinese cooking. Don't worry; the final taste is not fishy and the powerful scent fades on cooking. There is no substitute, but if you cannot find it, replace it with soy sauce.

Sauce

1 cup	light coconut milk	250 mL
1 tbsp	packed brown sugar	15 mL
1 tbsp	reduced-sodium fish sauce or soy sauce	15 mL
2 tsp	cornstarch	10 mL

Shrimp

	Vegetable cooking spray	
¼	red onion, chopped	¼
2	bell peppers (any color), chopped	2
1 tsp	red curry paste (or to taste)	5 mL
8 oz	shrimp, peeled and deveined	250 g

1. *Sauce:* In a small bowl, whisk together coconut milk, brown sugar, fish sauce and cornstarch.

2. *Shrimp:* Heat a large skillet over medium heat. Spray with vegetable cooking spray. Sauté red onion until just soft, about 5 minutes. Add bell peppers and curry paste; cook until peppers are slightly soft, about 5 minutes. Add sauce and shrimp; bring to a boil. Reduce heat, cover and simmer for 5 minutes or until shrimp are pink and opaque.

This recipe courtesy of dietitian Heather Barnes.

Nutrients
PER SERVING

Calories	275
Fat	10 g
Carbohydrate	28 g
Fiber	2 g
Protein	20 g

Linguine with Chile Shrimp

Shrimp is an excellent source of antioxidants, anti-inflammatory nutrients and omega-3 fatty acids. In addition, shrimp are a great low-calorie protein source.

Tip

The longer you cook the chile pepper, the less heat it has. Removing the seeds also helps to reduce the spiciness.

Variation

If you cannot find arugula, substitute baby spinach.

8 oz	linguine	250 g
1 tbsp	olive oil	15 mL
2	cloves garlic, minced	2
½	red bell pepper, chopped	½
14 to 16	shrimp, peeled and deveined	14 to 16
½	small red chile pepper, seeded and finely chopped (or a pinch of hot pepper flakes)	½
2 tbsp	soft margarine	30 mL
1 tbsp	freshly squeezed lemon juice	15 mL
	Handful arugula	

1. Cook linguine according to package directions until al dente (tender to the bite). Drain.

2. Meanwhile, in a large skillet, heat olive oil over medium heat. Sauté garlic for a few seconds, being careful not to burn it. Add red pepper; sauté for about 2 minutes or until it begins to soften. Add shrimp and chile pepper; cook for 1 to 2 minutes, or until shrimp are pink and opaque. Remove from heat and add margarine and linguine; toss to coat.

3. Serve immediately, drizzled with lemon juice and topped with arugula.

This recipe courtesy of dietitian Samantha Thiessen.

Nutrients
PER SERVING

Calories	335
Fat	11 g
Carbohydrate	45 g
Fiber	3 g
Protein	14 g

Asparagus, Lemon and Dill Shrimp Linguine

Light, refreshing flavors complement whole wheat linguine perfectly in this delightful seafood pasta dish.

Tips

If you can't find spot prawns, use medium shrimp (size 31 to 35).

Cooking the asparagus with the pasta saves a pot.

Variation

Use 2 cups (500 mL) chopped broccoli instead of asparagus.

8 oz	whole wheat linguine	250 g
8 oz	asparagus spears, trimmed and cut into 2-inch (5 cm) pieces	250 g
1 tbsp	canola oil	15 mL
3	shallots, sliced	3
3	cloves garlic, minced	3
1 cup	dry white wine	250 mL
	Grated zest and juice of 1 lemon	
1	package (12 oz/340 g) wild British Columbia spot prawns, peeled and deveined	1
½ cup	freshly grated Parmesan cheese	125 mL
¼ cup	chopped fresh dill	60 mL

1. In a large pot of boiling salted water, cook pasta according to package directions until al dente, adding asparagus for the last 3 minutes of cooking time. Drain and transfer to a large serving bowl.

2. Meanwhile, in a large skillet, heat oil over medium heat. Sauté shallots for 3 to 4 minutes or until softened. Add garlic and sauté for 30 seconds. Add wine, lemon zest and lemon juice; bring to a boil, stirring. Stir in prawns and simmer for 2 to 3 minutes or until pink and opaque.

3. Pour prawn mixture over pasta mixture and stir to combine. Sprinkle with Parmesan and dill.

This recipe courtesy of dietitian Heather McColl.

Nutrients	
PER SERVING	
Calories	280
Fat	6 g
Carbohydrate	33 g
Fiber	4 g
Protein	21 g

Shrimp and Mussels with Couscous

Here's a dish that is as delicious as it is easy to prepare! The couscous makes a great accompaniment — and it's ready in minutes.

Tips

Mussels should be rinsed in several changes of cold water to rid them of any grit. If still intact, the beard from the outer mussel shells should be removed by scrubbing with a hard brush prior to cooking. Inspect mussels before cooking and discard any with shells that are broken or any that do not close when tapped: these are not safe to eat. Likewise, discard any that have not opened after cooking.

Couscous is made from hard durum semolina wheat. It is popular in Middle Eastern cooking, particularly in Moroccan cuisine.

Nutrients PER SERVING	
Calories	390
Fat	5 g
Carbohydrate	69 g
Fiber	5 g
Protein	18 g

1 tbsp	olive oil	15 mL
1 cup	sliced leeks (green and white parts)	250 mL
1/2 cup	diced carrots	125 mL
1	can (19 oz/540 mL) stewed tomatoes	1
1 tsp	minced garlic	5 mL
1 cup	green bell pepper strips	250 mL
1 lb	fresh mussels, cleaned and debearded	500 g
1 1/2 cups	quick-cooking couscous	375 mL
12	cooked large shrimp	12

1. In a large saucepan or Dutch oven, heat oil over medium-high heat. Add leeks and sauté for 2 to 3 minutes. Add carrots, tomatoes and garlic; bring to a boil. Cover, reduce heat and simmer for 10 minutes.

2. Add green pepper strips and mussels; cook, covered, for about 5 minutes or until mussels have opened. Discard any mussels that haven't opened.

3. Meanwhile, cook couscous according to package directions.

4. Add shrimp to mussel mixture; cook for 2 minutes or until heated through. Serve over couscous.

This recipe courtesy of Johanne Trepanier.

Vegetarian Main Dishes

Big-Batch Italian Tomato Master Sauce

Makes 12 cups (3 L)

This Italian master sauce makes a great base for many pasta dishes. Use on pasta alone, or with beans, vegetables and protein added; as a base for minestrone soup; or to replace commercial tomato sauce in any of your recipes.

Tips

Stovetop Method: If you don't have a slow cooker, you can still make the sauce by adjusting the method slightly. Sauté the onions and garlic in a large pot, then add all of the other ingredients and bring to a boil. Reduce heat, cover and simmer, stirring occasionally, for 4 hours, until flavor is developed.

If you prefer a thicker sauce, purée it slightly.

- **Large (minimum 6-quart) slow cooker**

3 tbsp	olive oil	45 mL
6	cloves garlic, minced	6
1	large Spanish onion, finely chopped	1
1 tsp	salt, divided	5 mL
4	cans (each 28 oz/796 mL) whole tomatoes, with juice, chopped	4
4	sprigs fresh basil, divided	4
1 tsp	dried oregano	5 mL
½ tsp	freshly ground black pepper	2 mL
	Granulated sugar (optional)	

1. In a large skillet, heat olive oil over medium-high heat. Add garlic and onion; season lightly with some of the salt. Sauté until lightly browned, about 5 minutes.

2. Transfer sautéed vegetables to slow cooker. Stir in tomatoes, 3 of the basil sprigs, oregano, pepper and the remaining salt. Cover and cook on Low for 8 hours, until flavor is developed. If sauce is too thin, near the end of the cooking time increase to High and keep lid slightly open until sauce thickens. Discard basil sprigs.

3. Chop the remaining basil sprig and add to sauce. Taste and season with salt and pepper, if desired. Add sugar if sauce is too tart.

This recipe courtesy of Eileen Campbell.

Nutrients
PER 6 TBSP (90 ML)

Calories	34
Fat	1 g
Carbohydrate	5 g
Fiber	1 g
Protein	1 g

Chickpea Curry

Here's a nutrient-rich recipe that is kind to the heart and waistline.

Tips

Cooked chickpeas provide a whopping 5.5 g of fiber per ¾ cup (175 mL).

This curry is delicious inside a whole wheat pita.

2 tbsp	vegetable oil	30 mL
¾ cup	diced onion	175 mL
1 tbsp	curry powder	15 mL
1 to 2 tbsp	all-purpose flour (or 1 tbsp/15 mL cornstarch)	15 to 30 mL
1 cup	water (approx.)	250 mL
⅔ cup	diced red bell pepper	150 mL
⅔ cup	diced yellow bell pepper	150 mL
1 cup	diced zucchini	250 mL
¾ cup	diced butternut squash	175 mL
1	can (19 oz/540 mL) chickpeas, drained and rinsed (about 2 cups/500 mL)	1
½ cup	vegetable broth	125 mL
½ cup	snow peas (optional)	125 mL
¼ cup	finely chopped fresh parsley (or 1 tbsp/15 mL dried)	60 mL

1. In a large skillet, heat oil over medium heat. Sauté onions until softened, about 5 minutes. Stir in curry powder. Sprinkle with 1 tbsp (15 mL) flour. Add water, stirring constantly to prevent lumping.

2. Add red and yellow peppers, zucchini and squash; bring to a boil. Cook, stirring often, for 10 minutes, adding more water if sauce is too thick. (If it's too thin, add the remaining flour, mixed with a little water.)

3. Add chickpeas and broth; reduce heat and simmer for 10 minutes, until chickpeas are heated through. Add snow peas (if using) and parsley just before serving.

This recipe courtesy of dietitian Lindsay Mandryk.

Nutrients PER SERVING	
Calories	169
Fat	6 g
Carbohydrate	26 g
Fiber	5 g
Protein	5 g

Vegetarian Chili

A fiber-rich vegetarian version of the classic.

Tips

If you cannot find Mexican-flavored vegetarian ground round, use regular vegetarian ground round and add 2 tbsp (30 mL) chili powder.

Freeze this dish in meal-sized portions so you can have a hot, healthy meal anytime.

Serve with half a bagel and a glass of milk.

Variation

Substitute a 12-oz (341 mL) can of peaches-and-cream corn, drained, for the carrots.

1 tbsp	vegetable oil	15 mL
2	cloves garlic, diced	2
½ cup	diced red onion	125 mL
1	package (12 oz/340 g) Mexican-flavored vegetarian ground round	1
1 cup	diced green bell pepper	250 mL
2	cans (each 19 oz/540 mL) diced tomatoes (about 4¾ cups/1.175 L)	2
1	can (19 oz/540 mL) red kidney beans, drained and rinsed (about 2 cups/500 mL)	1
1 cup	grated carrots	250 mL
1 tbsp	dried parsley	15 mL
1 tsp	hot pepper sauce	5 mL
	Freshly ground black pepper	
½ cup	shredded Cheddar cheese	125 mL

1. In a large skillet, heat oil over medium heat. Sauté garlic and red onion until softened, about 5 minutes. Add ground round, breaking it apart with a wooden spoon to prevent clumps; sauté for 2 to 3 minutes or until evenly heated. Add green pepper and sauté for 2 to 3 minutes. Add tomatoes, beans, carrots, parsley, hot pepper sauce and pepper to taste; cook, stirring occasionally, for 10 minutes or until beans are heated through.

2. Ladle into serving bowls and sprinkle with cheese.

This recipe courtesy of dietitian Lindsay Mandryk.

Nutrients
PER SERVING

Calories	194
Fat	6 g
Carbohydrate	20 g
Fiber	7 g
Protein	15 g

Easy Black Beans

This spicy recipe is great for those rushed days when you're not very organized and are wondering what to make for supper as you drive home. When you are more organized, plan ahead and soak some beans instead of using canned.

Tips

If your family doesn't like heat, leave out the chipotle pepper.

Serve with stir-fried kale and steamed basmati rice.

1 tsp	vegetable oil	5 mL
1	small onion, chopped	1
1	can (19 oz/540 mL) black beans, drained and rinsed (about 2 cups/500 mL)	1
1½ cups	water	375 mL
½ cup	tomato paste	125 mL
1	chipotle pepper in adobo sauce	1
1	bay leaf	1
1 tsp	ground cumin	5 mL
2 tbsp	chopped fresh cilantro (optional)	30 mL

1. In a large skillet, heat oil over medium heat. Sauté onion until softened, about 5 minutes. Stir in beans, water, tomato paste, chipotle pepper, bay leaf and cumin; bring to a boil. Reduce heat and simmer for 15 minutes or until slightly thickened. Discard the chipotle and bay leaf. (If you leave the chipotle in, the dish will be too spicy!)

2. Ladle into bowls and garnish with cilantro, if desired.

This recipe courtesy of dietitian Chantal Saad Haddad.

Nutrients
PER SERVING

Calories	145
Fat	2 g
Carbohydrate	26 g
Fiber	9 g
Protein	8 g

Quick and Easy Lentil Tacos

Even some meat lovers will make this dish their go-to taco recipe. It's faster and cheaper and has easier cleanup than meat tacos.

Tips

This dish is a breeze to prepare if one person gets the lentil mixture ready and sets the table while another chops the veggies and shreds the cheese.

You can use 1 can (19 oz/540 mL) lentils, drained and rinsed, instead of cooked lentils.

Variation

To make a taco salad, spoon the lentil filling on top of a bed of lettuce and tomato, then sprinkle with cheese and garnish with baked tortilla chips.

1½ cups	cooked green lentils	375 mL
2 tbsp	finely minced red onion	30 mL
2 tbsp	finely minced red bell pepper	30 mL
¼ cup	salsa	60 mL
4	taco shells	4
¾ cup	finely shredded romaine or iceberg lettuce	175 mL
¾ cup	finely diced plum (Roma) tomatoes	175 mL
½ cup	shredded regular or light Cheddar cheese	125 mL
½ cup	light sour cream (optional)	125 mL
1	avocado, cubed (optional)	1
½ cup	sliced black olives (optional)	125 mL

1. In a medium saucepan, over medium heat, combine lentils, onion, red pepper and salsa; cook, stirring often, for 3 to 4 minutes or until bubbling and hot.

2. Fill each taco shell with one-fourth of the lentil mixture, lettuce, tomatoes and cheese. If desired, top with sour cream, avocado and olives.

This recipe courtesy of dietitian Amanda Beales.

Nutrients
PER SERVING

Calories	219
Fat	8 g
Carbohydrate	27 g
Fiber	5 g
Protein	12 g

Portobello Mushroom Burgers with Cheese Filling

Makes 4 servings

Here's another lower-calorie reason to eat vegetarian.

Tips

Adding the chopped mushroom stems improves the texture of the cheese mixture.

The cheese mixture also makes a great veggie dip.

- Preheat barbecue grill to medium
- Food processor

4	large portobello mushrooms	4
2 tsp	olive oil	10 mL
2	cloves garlic, minced	2
2 cups	tightly packed fresh spinach leaves	500 mL
2 tbsp	chopped fresh basil	30 mL
1 cup	2% cottage cheese	250 mL
1/4 cup	freshly grated Parmesan cheese	60 mL
4	4-inch (10 cm) whole wheat pitas, split open	4
	Roasted red pepper slices (optional)	

1. Wipe mushroom caps with a damp paper towel and gently twist off stems. Coarsely chop stems and set aside. Using the edge of a spoon, gently scrape off and discard the dark gills from the caps.

2. Brush both sides of mushroom caps with oil and place on preheated grill. Grill, turning once, for 2 to 3 minutes per side or until lightly browned on both sides. Set aside.

3. In food processor, combine mushroom stems, garlic, spinach, basil, cottage cheese and Parmesan; process until uniformly smooth but not puréed.

4. Place 1 grilled mushroom cap, rounded side down, on a pita half and fill with one-quarter of the cheese mixture. Top with the other pita half. Garnish with roasted peppers (if using).

This recipe courtesy of Lynn Dowling.

Nutrients
PER SERVING

Calories	278
Fat	7 g
Carbohydrate	39 g
Fiber	6 g
Protein	19 g

Eggplant Lasagna

This vegetarian entrée features a surprising filling that will delight your family.

Tips

If you cannot get 9 slices from the eggplant, cut larger slices in half lengthwise to obtain the desired number.

If you are trying to get picky eaters to eat more vegetables, use half lasagna sheets and half eggplant slices, then slowly add more eggplant over time.

The hummus mixture also makes a delicious dip.

Variation

Use 3 cooked whole wheat lasagna sheets instead of the eggplant.

- **Preheat oven to 400°F (200°C)**
- **Baking sheet, lightly greased**
- **9-inch (23 cm) square glass baking dish, lightly greased**

1	eggplant (about 1 lb/500 g)	1
½ tsp	freshly ground black pepper	2 mL
¼ tsp	salt	1 mL
1 cup	drained thawed chopped frozen spinach	250 mL
1 cup	tomato sauce	250 mL
1 cup	2% cottage cheese	250 mL
½ cup	spicy red pepper hummus	125 mL
2 tbsp	freshly grated Parmesan cheese	30 mL

1. Peel eggplant and cut lengthwise into 9 thin slices. Season both sides with pepper and salt. Place on prepared baking sheet and roast in preheated oven, turning once, for 15 minutes or until lightly browned. Set aside.

2. Meanwhile, in a small bowl, combine spinach and tomato sauce.

3. In another small bowl, combine cottage cheese and hummus.

4. Spread ¼ cup (60 mL) of the tomato sauce mixture over bottom of prepared baking dish. Arrange 3 eggplant slices on top. Spread with one-third of the cottage cheese mixture. Add 2 more layers of sauce, eggplant and cheese. Pour the remaining sauce over top and sprinkle with Parmesan.

5. Bake in preheated oven for 20 minutes or until cheese is golden and lasagna is heated through. Let stand for 10 minutes before cutting.

This recipe courtesy of Lorna Salgado.

Nutrients
PER SERVING

Calories	210
Fat	9 g
Carbohydrate	21 g
Fiber	5 g
Protein	13 g

Moroccan Vegetable Tagine

This colorful and healthy blend of vegetables scented with saffron, lemon and parsley works beautifully served with steamed whole wheat couscous or brown rice.

Tips

Nothing can really substitute for the flavor of saffron, but the pretty yellow-orange color it creates can be mimicked with ½ tsp (2 mL) ground turmeric.

There are about 2⅓ cups (575 mL) of diced tomatoes in a 19-oz (540 mL) can and about 2 cups (500 mL) of drained chickpeas in a 19-oz can.

Add whole wheat couscous and serve fresh fruit and yogurt or cheese for dessert.

1 tbsp	olive oil	15 mL
2	onions, chopped	2
2	cloves garlic, finely chopped	2
2	Yukon gold potatoes, peeled and cubed	2
2	large carrots, cut into short sticks	2
½	large sweet potato, peeled and cut into short sticks	½
1 tbsp	grated gingerroot	15 mL
1 tsp	ground cumin	5 mL
1 tsp	ground cinnamon	5 mL
1	can (19 oz/540 mL) diced tomatoes	1
1	can (19 oz/540 mL) chickpeas, drained and rinsed	1
4 cups	vegetable broth	1 L
Pinch	saffron strands (optional)	Pinch
¼ cup	chopped fresh parsley	60 mL
	Juice of 1 lemon	
	Salt and freshly ground black pepper	
2 tbsp	hot pepper sauce (optional)	30 mL

1. In a large saucepan, heat oil over medium-high heat. Add onions, garlic, potatoes, carrots, sweet potato, ginger, cumin and cinnamon; cook, stirring often, for 10 minutes.

2. Stir in tomatoes; cook for 2 minutes. Stir in chickpeas, broth and saffron (if using); bring to a boil. Reduce heat, cover and simmer for 30 minutes, until vegetables are just tender. Stir in parsley and lemon juice. Season to taste with salt and pepper. Stir in hot sauce (if using).

This recipe courtesy of dietitian Donna Bottrell.

Nutrients
PER SERVING

Calories	175
Fat	3 g
Carbohydrate	34 g
Fiber	5 g
Protein	5 g

Vegetable Moussaka

This is a great lower-fat vegetarian version of a Greek classic. The rich cream sauce normally used in moussaka has been replaced with a tofu mixture that gives all the taste with a fraction of the fat!

Tips

Eggplant is a source of soluble fiber.

To vary the flavors in this tasty dish and transform it into a great party pleaser, add grilled peppers and zucchini to the eggplant layer.

- **Preheat oven to 350°F (180°C)**
- **Baking sheets, greased**
- **Food processor**
- **13- by 9-inch (33 by 23 cm) baking pan, greased**

2	eggplants	2
	Salt	
1	onion, chopped	1
1	clove garlic, minced	1
1	can (19 oz/540 mL) chickpeas, drained and rinsed	1
1	can (28 oz/796 mL) tomatoes	1
1 tbsp	dried oregano	15 mL
1 tbsp	dried basil	15 mL
1/2 tsp	ground cinnamon	2 mL
1/2 tsp	freshly ground black pepper	2 mL
1/4 cup	freshly grated Parmesan cheese	60 mL

Topping

1 lb	tofu	500 g
1	onion, quartered	1
2	egg whites	2
Pinch	ground nutmeg	Pinch

1. Slice eggplants lengthwise into 1/4-inch (0.5 cm) thick slices; sprinkle with salt. Drain in colander for 30 minutes. Place on prepared baking sheets and bake in preheated oven for 15 minutes. Turn and bake for 15 minutes longer.

2. In a nonstick skillet sprayed with nonstick cooking spray, cook onion and garlic, stirring, for 2 minutes. Add chickpeas, mashing slightly. Stir in tomatoes, oregano, basil, cinnamon, pepper and 1/2 tsp (2 mL) salt; bring to a boil. Reduce heat and simmer, uncovered, for 20 minutes, stirring occasionally. Process in food processor until mixture resembles coarse meal.

Nutrients
PER SERVING

Calories	187
Fat	5 g
Carbohydrate	26 g
Fiber	6 g
Protein	12 g

3. In prepared baking pan, layer half of the eggplant, then all of the chickpea mixture, half of the Parmesan, then remaining eggplant.

4. *Topping:* Purée ingredients for topping; spread over moussaka. Sprinkle with remaining cheese. Bake in preheated oven for 30 minutes.

This recipe courtesy of chef Mark Mogensen and dietitian Marsha Rosen.

Spaghetti Squash with Mushrooms

Makes 6 servings

Spaghetti squash, which is most readily available from August to November, looks just like golden strands of spaghetti yet tastes like squash when cooked. Since spaghetti squash acts like both pasta and vegetable, you can serve it with your favorite spaghetti sauce.

Tips

Spaghetti squash is easily recognized by its oblong shape and pale to bright yellow skin. It bakes and microwaves quite easily.

To keep the strands intact, be sure to cut squash in half lengthwise.

Serve this dish over brown rice for a more substantial meal.

- **Preheat oven to 350°F (180°C)**
- **Baking sheet**

1	spaghetti squash (about 3½ lbs/1.5 kg)	1
2 cups	sliced mushrooms	500 mL
1	green onion, sliced	1
1	small stalk celery, chopped	1
2 cups	chopped tomatoes (4 small)	500 mL
2 tbsp	margarine	30 mL
2 tbsp	all-purpose flour	30 mL
1 cup	2% milk	250 mL
½ cup	shredded Cheddar cheese	125 mL
1 tsp	dried oregano	5 mL
½ tsp	garlic powder	2 mL
½ tsp	salt	2 mL
¼ tsp	freshly ground black pepper	1 mL
	Freshly grated low-fat Parmesan cheese	

1. Cut squash in half lengthwise. Bake cut side down on a baking sheet in preheated oven for 25 to 30 minutes or boil, cut side down and covered, in 2 inches (5 cm) of water for about 20 minutes.

2. In a skillet over medium-high heat, cook mushrooms, onion, celery and tomatoes in margarine for about 5 minutes or until tender. Stir in flour; gradually add milk. Cook, stirring constantly, until thickened. Stir in Cheddar cheese and seasonings until cheese is melted.

3. Pour sauce over squash; sprinkle with Parmesan cheese and serve.

This recipe courtesy of Marlyn Ambrose-Chase.

Nutrients
PER SERVING

Calories	163
Fat	8 g
Carbohydrate	18 g
Fiber	4 g
Protein	6 g

Butternut Squash, Spinach and Feta Frittata

A versatile recipe for breakfast or dinner. You choose.

Tips

Butternut squash can be difficult to peel. To make the task easier, first cut the squash in half crosswise, to create two flat surfaces. Place each squash half on its flat surface and use a sharp utility knife to remove the tough peel.

Serve with a green salad or a steamed green vegetable such as peas, beans or edamame. To boost the protein in this meal, sprinkle the salad or vegetable with toasted nuts or seeds.

In a frittata, the ingredients are mixed in with the eggs; in an omelet they are folded inside cooked eggs.

- Preheat oven to 400°F (200°C)
- 13- by 9-inch (33 by 23 cm) glass baking dish, lightly greased

1	butternut squash, peeled and cubed (4 to 5 cups/1 to 1.25 L)	1
1	package (10 oz/300 g) frozen chopped spinach, thawed and drained	1
1½ cups	cubed peeled potatoes	375 mL
¾ cup	thinly sliced red onion	175 mL
8	eggs	8
½ cup	1% milk	125 mL
	Freshly ground black pepper	
1 cup	shredded Cheddar cheese	250 mL
½ cup	crumbled feta cheese	125 mL

1. Place squash in a large microwave-safe bowl and cover with plastic wrap, leaving a corner open to vent. Microwave on High for about 5 minutes or until fork-tender. Drain off excess liquid. Gently stir in spinach, potatoes and red onion. Spread in prepared baking dish.

2. In a bowl, whisk together eggs and milk. Season to taste with pepper. Pour over vegetables and stir gently to distribute. Sprinkle evenly with Cheddar and feta.

3. Bake in preheated oven for 35 to 40 minutes or until eggs are set.

This recipe courtesy of dietitian Lindsay Mandryk.

Nutrients
PER SERVING

Calories	151
Fat	8 g
Carbohydrate	12 g
Fiber	2 g
Protein	9 g

Potato-Crusted Zucchini, Carrot and Smoked Cheddar Quiche

The delicate vegetable flavors in this quiche are enhanced by the smokiness of the cheese.

Tips

It's important to parboil the potatoes to soften them and keep them from turning brown, but make sure not to overcook them in step 1, or they will break apart.

Smoked cheese derives its flavor from light smoking using wood from a fruitwood tree, such as apple or cherry. Applewood smoking lends Cheddar cheese a sweet, subtle smoky flavor.

Variations

For some heat, add ¼ tsp (1 mL) cayenne pepper or ½ tsp (2 mL) hot pepper sauce to the vegetables.

For a slightly different flavor, add ½ tsp (2 mL) ground cumin to the vegetables.

- Preheat oven to 350°F (180°C)
- 9-inch (23 cm) glass pie plate, greased

12 oz	russet potatoes, cut into ⅛-inch (3 mm) slices	375 g
1 tsp	canola oil	5 mL
2 cups	chopped zucchini	500 mL
1 cup	thinly sliced carrot coins	250 mL
⅓ cup	finely chopped onion	75 mL
1	clove garlic, minced	1
½ tsp	freshly ground black pepper	2 mL
Pinch	ground nutmeg	Pinch
4	eggs	4
1 cup	shredded applewood-smoked Cheddar cheese	250 mL
½ cup	1% to 2% milk	125 mL

1. Bring a medium saucepan of water to a boil over high heat. Add potatoes, reduce heat and simmer for 7 minutes or until fork-tender. Drain. Line bottom of prepared pie plate with enough slices to cover, overlapping slightly (you may not need all of the potato slices).

2. Meanwhile, in a skillet, heat oil over medium heat. Sauté zucchini, carrots and onion for 4 to 5 minutes or until softened. Add garlic, pepper and nutmeg; sauté for 30 seconds. Spoon vegetables over potatoes.

3. In a medium bowl, whisk eggs until blended. Stir in cheese and milk. Pour evenly over vegetable mixture.

4. Bake in preheated oven for 30 minutes or until set in the center. Let cool for 10 to 15 minutes. Cut into 6 wedges.

This recipe courtesy of dietitian Heather McColl.

Nutrients PER SERVING	
Calories	203
Fat	11 g
Carbohydrate	16 g
Fiber	2 g
Protein	11 g

Teriyaki Tofu Stir-Fry

This recipe is great for someone who is trying tofu for the first time. It's easy to prepare and very tasty.

Tips

Use any vegetables you like or have on hand, such as broccoli and cauliflower, snow peas, green beans, mushrooms, tomatoes or thinly sliced carrots.

Be sure to do your preparation — washing, chopping and dicing — ahead of time so that everything comes together when you are actually at the stove.

Teriyaki sauce is quite high in salt. So if you need to limit your salt intake, replace the teriyaki sauce with sodium-reduced soy sauce.

1⅓ cups	diced firm tofu	325 mL
½ cup	teriyaki sauce	125 mL
1 tsp	brown sugar	5 mL
1 tsp	cornstarch	5 mL
1 tbsp	water	15 mL
2 tsp	olive oil	10 mL
½ cup	finely chopped onion	125 mL
1 cup	finely chopped green bell peppers	250 mL
1 cup	finely chopped red bell peppers	250 mL
1 tsp	minced garlic	5 mL
1 tsp	grated gingerroot	5 mL
2 cups	roughly chopped vegetables (see tip, at left)	500 mL
3 cups	cooked rice	750 mL
1 to 2 tbsp	chopped fresh cilantro or parsley (optional)	15 to 30 mL

1. In a medium bowl, gently toss tofu with teriyaki sauce and brown sugar until well coated. Cover and refrigerate for 10 minutes or for up to several hours.

2. In a small bowl, whisk together cornstarch and water. Set aside.

3. In a large nonstick skillet, heat oil over medium-high heat. Add onion, green peppers, red peppers, garlic and ginger; stir-fry for 3 minutes. Stir in vegetables of your choice and stir-fry for 3 to 4 minutes or until vegetables are tender-crisp.

4. Add tofu mixture and cornstarch mixture. Stir for 3 to 4 minutes or until thickened and heated through. Serve over rice. Sprinkle with cilantro, if using.

This recipe courtesy of dietitian Lorraine Fullum-Bouchard.

Nutrients
PER SERVING

Calories	287
Fat	5 g
Carbohydrate	49 g
Fiber	3 g
Protein	12 g

Tofu Patties

Makes 6 servings

This is a great way to prepare tofu. For children, make mini patties and place on whole-grain dinner rolls with their choice of condiments.

Tips

Look for tofu made with calcium. Look for "calcium sulfate" or "calcium chloride" in the ingredients list to make sure the tofu you are buying is a source of calcium.

Place on a multigrain bun and top with sliced tomato, leaf lettuce and a dab of your favorite mustard or salsa.

- **Preheat oven to 325°F (160°C)**
- **9-inch (23 cm) square baking pan, lightly greased**

10 oz	firm tofu, mashed	300 g
¾ cup	quick-cooking rolled oats	175 mL
2 tbsp	soy sauce	30 mL
½ tsp	dried basil	2 mL
½ tsp	dried oregano	2 mL
½ tsp	garlic powder	2 mL
½ tsp	onion powder	2 mL
	Salt and freshly ground black pepper	

1. In a medium bowl, combine tofu, oats, soy sauce, basil, oregano, garlic powder, onion powder, and salt and pepper to taste. Knead for a few minutes. Shape into 1-inch (2.5 cm) thick patties and place in prepared pan.

2. Bake in preheated oven for 20 to 25 minutes or until lightly browned.

This recipe courtesy of dietitian Sue Minicucci.

Nutrients
PER SERVING

Calories	83
Fat	3 g
Carbohydrate	10 g
Fiber	2 g
Protein	6 g

Side Dishes

Roasted Lemon Asparagus

This dish has loads of tang from the fresh lemon juice and zest, so pucker up!

Tips

The baking time will vary depending on the width of the asparagus spears. Check occasionally for doneness.

For an extra flourish, sprinkle the cooked asparagus with 2 tbsp (30 mL) freshly grated low-fat Parmesan cheese.

Cook asparagus soon after you purchase it or the natural sugars will quickly turn to starch and the texture will be woody.

You can also grill the asparagus, either on the baking sheet or in a grill basket on a barbecue grill preheated to medium-high.

- **Preheat oven to 350°F (180°C)**
- **Rimmed baking sheet, lined with foil**

1	bunch asparagus (about 1 lb/500 g), ends trimmed	1
1	lemon	1
2	cloves garlic, minced	2
2 tbsp	olive oil	30 mL
¼ tsp	salt	1 mL
¼ tsp	freshly ground black pepper	1 mL

1. Spread asparagus on prepared baking sheet. Grate zest and squeeze juice from ½ lemon into a small bowl. Stir in garlic, oil, salt and pepper. Pour over asparagus and shake pan to ensure each spear is coated.

2. Cut the remaining lemon half into slices and place among asparagus spears.

3. Bake in preheated oven, turning once, for 10 to 12 minutes or until lightly browned and tender-crisp.

This recipe courtesy of dietitian Honey Bloomberg.

Nutrients
PER SERVING

Calories	83
Fat	7 g
Carbohydrate	5 g
Fiber	2 g
Protein	2 g

Green Beans with Tomato Sauce

Green beans pack a nutritional punch!

Tip

Green beans contain soluble fiber and a small amount of chromium.

1 tbsp	garlic-infused olive oil	15 mL
4	green onions, sliced	4
1	can (19 oz/540 mL) diced tomatoes, with juice	1
1 cup	water	250 mL
1 lb	green beans, ends trimmed	500 g
2 tbsp	chopped fresh dill	30 mL
	Salt and freshly ground black pepper	

1. In a medium skillet, heat oil over medium heat. Cook green onions, stirring, for 3 to 5 minutes or until tender. Add tomatoes with juice and simmer, stirring occasionally, for about 15 minutes to blend the flavors.

2. Meanwhile, in a large saucepan, bring water to a boil over high heat. Add beans and dill. Reduce heat to medium, cover and cook for about 25 minutes or until beans are tender. Drain and stir into tomato sauce. Season to taste with salt and pepper.

Nutrients
PER SERVING

Calories	70
Fat	3 g
Carbohydrate	12 g
Fiber	4 g
Protein	2 g

Braised Red Cabbage

Did you know red cabbage contains almost twice the vitamin C of green cabbage? In addition to vitamin C, it's packed with fiber, vitamin K, vitamin B$_6$, potassium and manganese.

Tip

Refrigerate the cooked cabbage for 24 hours, then reheat it in a pot over medium-low heat, stirring often, until heated through. This technique produces the most flavorful dish.

Variation

Use ground allspice instead of ground cloves.

2 tsp	canola oil	10 mL
1 cup	chopped onion	250 mL
1	apple, peeled and chopped	1
8 cups	shredded red cabbage (1 small to medium head)	2 L
¾ cup	packed brown sugar	175 mL
1 tsp	ground cloves	5 mL
½ tsp	salt	2 mL
½ tsp	freshly ground black pepper	2 mL
½ cup	cider vinegar	125 mL

1. In a Dutch oven with a tight-fitting lid, heat oil over medium heat. Sauté onion for 3 to 4 minutes or until softened. Add apple and sauté for 1 minute or until softened.

2. Stir in cabbage, brown sugar, cloves, salt, pepper and vinegar; increase heat to medium-high and bring to a boil. Reduce heat to low, cover and simmer, stirring occasionally, for about 30 minutes or until cabbage is soft. Serve warm or transfer to a bowl and refrigerate until chilled.

This recipe courtesy of dietitian Corinne Eisenbraun.

Nutrients
PER SERVING

Calories	135
Fat	1 g
Carbohydrate	30 g
Fiber	2 g
Protein	1 g

Ginger Carrots

MMMmmmm good — a delicious way to enjoy carrots.

Tip

Use the side of a spoon to scrape off the skin of gingerroot before chopping or grating. Gingerroot keeps well in the freezer for up to 3 months and can be grated from frozen.

4 cups	chopped carrots	1 L
½ cup	vegetable or chicken broth	125 mL
2 tsp	minced gingerroot	10 mL
1 tsp	minced garlic	5 mL
1 tsp	packed brown sugar	5 mL
¼ tsp	freshly squeezed lemon juice	1 mL

1. In a large saucepan, combine carrots, broth, ginger, garlic, brown sugar and lemon juice. Bring to a boil, then reduce heat, cover and simmer for about 20 minutes or until carrots are tender-crisp and liquid is absorbed.

This recipe courtesy of dietitian Roberta Lowcay.

Nutrients
PER SERVING

Calories	34
Fat	0 g
Carbohydrate	8 g
Fiber	2 g
Protein	1 g

Spinach Fancy

Makes 5 servings

No one will have to tell you to eat your spinach anymore! You will be more than willing to enjoy this tasty dish, which is particularly good with fish.

Tips

Use fresh herbs to replace any of the dried herbs in this recipe, but double or triple the amounts, as the drying process intensifies the flavor of herbs.

Like all dark leafy greens, spinach is a source of vitamin A, folate and non-heme iron. When consuming foods that contain iron, avoid drinking caffeinated beverages, such as coffee, tea or cola, for at least an hour, as caffeine can reduce the body's ability to absorb iron.

1	package (10 oz/300 g) fresh spinach	1
3 tbsp	raisins	45 mL
Pinch	dried mint	Pinch
Pinch	ground fennel	Pinch
Pinch	dried oregano	Pinch
1 tbsp	soft margarine	15 mL
2 tbsp	water	30 mL
1 tsp	freshly squeezed lemon juice	5 mL
½ tsp	salt	2 mL
Pinch	freshly ground black pepper	Pinch
	Lemon slices	

1. Wash spinach and dry thoroughly; remove stems and chop leaves.

2. In a large skillet over medium heat, cook raisins, mint, fennel and oregano in margarine. Add spinach and water; cover and steam for 2 to 3 minutes or until wilted. Drain liquid. Sprinkle with lemon juice, salt and pepper; toss well. Serve with lemon slices.

This recipe courtesy of Martine Lortie.

Nutrients
PER SERVING

Calories	50
Fat	2 g
Carbohydrate	7 g
Fiber	1 g
Protein	2 g

Quick and Delicious Maple Squash

Squash is rich in vitamin A and fiber, and can easily be incorporated into any meal plan.

Tips

Microwave ovens vary in their capacity and power. Use a baking dish that fits easily inside. Cut the squash into smaller pieces, if necessary, or cook it one half at a time. Check the squash occasionally for doneness.

Butternut squash is one of the varieties classified as a winter squash (others include acorn and Hubbard). Winter squash are harvested in the late fall and can take as long as 3 months to ripen. They have tough outer skins that help them store well over the winter months.

Variation

Use 1 large buttercup or 2 medium acorn squash.

Nutrients PER SERVING	
Calories	97
Fat	1 g
Carbohydrate	22 g
Fiber	3 g
Protein	2 g

• **Large microwave-safe dish**

1	butternut squash	1
2 tbsp	pure maple syrup	30 mL
2 tsp	soft margarine	10 mL
½ tsp	freshly ground black pepper	2 mL
¼ tsp	salt	1 mL

1. Cut squash in half lengthwise. Scoop out and discard seeds and stringy pulp. Place squash, skin side down, in microwave-safe dish. Place 1 tbsp (15 mL) maple syrup and 1 tsp (5 mL) margarine in the hollow of each half.

2. Cover dish with plastic wrap, leaving one corner open for a vent, and microwave on High for 8 to 10 minutes or until fork-tender. Scoop squash out of skins into a serving dish. Sprinkle with pepper and salt.

This recipe courtesy of Erin Nelson.

Roasted Vegetables

With this recipe, all the chopping can be done in advance, then you can pop the dish in the oven when company arrives. Once the vegetables are roasted, arrange them on a serving platter or around a roasted chicken, beef roast or fillet of salmon.

Tips

This recipe is packed with soluble fiber!

For the herbs, try any combination of thyme, oregano, basil, dill, parsley, chives and rosemary — whatever suits your taste!

These vegetables can also be grilled in a vegetable basket on a lightly greased barbecue preheated to medium. Cook, turning once, until tender, about 10 minutes.

- Preheat oven to 325°F (160°C)
- 13- by 9-inch (33 by 23 cm) roasting pan or shallow casserole dish, lightly greased

2	bell peppers (any color)	2
2	parsnips, peeled	2
2	carrots	2
2	potatoes (unpeeled)	2
1	onion	1
1	zucchini	1
1	fennel bulb	1
3	cloves garlic	3
2 tbsp	vegetable oil	30 mL
2 tbsp	pure maple syrup or liquid honey	30 mL
1 tbsp	Dijon mustard	15 mL
2 tbsp	chopped fresh herbs (or 2 tsp/10 mL dried)	30 mL
	Freshly ground black pepper	

1. Chop peppers, parsnips, carrots, potatoes, onion, zucchini and fennel into bite-size chunks. Spread vegetables and garlic in prepared pan.

2. In a medium bowl, combine oil, maple syrup, mustard and herbs. Pour over vegetables and toss to coat. Sprinkle with pepper to taste.

3. Roast in preheated oven, tossing vegetables once, for 30 to 40 minutes or until fork-tender and golden.

This recipe courtesy of dietitian Dianna Bihun.

Nutrients
PER SERVING

Calories	150
Fat	4 g
Carbohydrate	28 g
Fiber	5 g
Protein	3 g

Dijon Mashed Potatoes

Makes 6 servings

It's time to enjoy a new spin on classic mashed potatoes. Potatoes are a good source of vitamin C and potassium.

Tip

Choose non-hydrogenated soft tub margarines. Check the label for nutrition information. The polyunsaturated and monounsaturated fats should add up to 6 g or more per 2-tsp (10 mL) serving.

2¾ lbs	round red potatoes, peeled and quartered	1.25 kg
3 tbsp	soft margarine	45 mL
⅔ cup	2% milk	150 mL
¼ cup	Dijon mustard	60 mL
	Salt and white pepper	

1. In a large pot of boiling salted water, cook potatoes for about 20 minutes or until tender. Drain well.

2. Return potatoes to pot and add margarine. Mash for about 1 minute or until smooth.

3. Stir in milk and mustard until blended. Season to taste with salt and pepper. Serve immediately.

Nutrients
PER SERVING

Calories	218
Fat	7 g
Carbohydrate	36 g
Fiber	4 g
Protein	5 g

Yam Fries

Makes 4 servings

These are a delicious and nutritious alternative to french fries.

Tip

Yams and sweet potatoes, while both sources of soluble fiber, are entirely different vegetables, with different colors, flavors and textures. The skin of yams ranges from brown to black, while the flesh can be off-white, pale yellow, purple or red.

- **Preheat oven to 425°F (220°C)**
- **2 rimmed baking sheets, lined with foil**

4	large yams, peeled	4
4 tsp	olive oil	20 mL
2 tsp	ground cumin	10 mL
2 tsp	ground coriander	10 mL
	Coarse salt and freshly ground black pepper	

1. Slice yams lengthwise into ½-inch (1 cm) thick slices. Cut slices into sticks and, as you work, immediately transfer to prepared baking sheets, drizzle with oil and roll sticks to coat all over (to prevent yams from turning black). Arrange coated sticks in single layer on sheets.

2. In a small bowl, combine cumin, coriander and salt and pepper to taste. Sprinkle over yams.

3. Bake in preheated oven, gently stirring and turning after 15 minutes, for 25 to 30 minutes or until crisp on the outside. Serve immediately.

Nutrients
PER SERVING

Calories	152
Fat	5 g
Carbohydrate	25 g
Fiber	4 g
Protein	3 g

Spinach Rice

This quick and easy dish provides a vegetable and a grain all in one tasty package.

2	packages (each 10 oz/300 g) frozen spinach, thawed	2
2 tbsp	olive oil	30 mL
4	bunches green onions, chopped	4
½ cup	chopped fresh dill	125 mL
½ cup	chopped fresh parsley	125 mL
1 cup	long-grain converted rice	250 mL
	Salt and freshly ground black pepper	
	Juice of 2 lemons	

1. In a colander, drain spinach, pressing out water with a fork. Set aside.

2. In a medium skillet, heat oil over medium heat. Sauté green onions for 3 to 5 minutes or until tender. Stir in spinach, dill and parsley and cook, stirring often, for about 10 minutes or until spinach is wilted. Remove from heat and set aside.

3. Cook rice for half the time specified in the package instructions.

4. Add rice and 2 cups (500 mL) water to spinach mixture and bring to a boil over high heat. Season to taste with salt and pepper. Reduce heat to medium, cover and cook, stirring occasionally, for 15 to 20 minutes or until rice is tender.

5. Remove from heat. Remove lid from skillet, replace with a tea towel and let stand for 10 to 15 minutes. Toss in lemon juice. Serve immediately.

Nutrients
PER SERVING

Calories	175
Fat	5 g
Carbohydrate	29 g
Fiber	1 g
Protein	4 g

Cornmeal Casserole

Makes 4 servings

This casserole is a delicious variation on Italian polenta.

Tips

If your cornmeal is "stone-ground," it will have a higher oil content than cornmeal that is processed by more modern methods. So be sure to store it in an airtight bag in the refrigerator (for up to 3 months) or in the freezer (for as long as 6 months).

Because sweet onions such as Spanish and Vidalia contain fewer sulfur compounds, they cause your eyes to water less when preparing. Use them for salads and in recipes with a delicate flavor such as this casserole.

Serve with yogurt and fresh berries for a complete meal.

- **Preheat oven to 350°F (180°C)**
- **4-cup (1 L) baking dish, lightly greased**

1	small onion, chopped	1
1	stalk celery, chopped	1
1 tbsp	margarine	15 mL
½ cup	yellow cornmeal	125 mL
½ tsp	salt	2 mL
½ tsp	granulated sugar	2 mL
Pinch	freshly ground black pepper	Pinch
2 cups	2% milk	500 mL
1	egg, well beaten	1

1. In a skillet over medium heat, cook onion and celery in margarine until golden. Stir in cornmeal and mix until coated. Add salt, sugar and pepper.

2. Scald milk; stir into cornmeal mixture. Cook over low heat until thickened; let cool. Stir in beaten egg and mix well. Spoon mixture into prepared baking dish. Bake, uncovered, in preheated oven for 35 to 40 minutes or until top is browned and casserole is set.

This recipe courtesy of Lydia Husak.

Nutrients
PER SERVING

Calories	170
Fat	7 g
Carbohydrate	20 g
Fiber	1 g
Protein	7 g

Desserts

Cinnamon Baked Pears

Here's an easy and delicious way to serve fruit. Try poaching peaches, nectarines, apples, fresh pineapple or oranges in this manner.

Tips

Most pears are shipped before they are fully ripe in order to avoid damage. If your pears are overly firm, store them in a cool place to ripen before using in this recipe.

For added fiber, leave the skin on pears, apples, peaches and nectarines when serving.

- **Preheat oven to 350°F (180°C)**
- **Glass baking dish**

4	pears	4
½ cup	blueberries	125 mL
½ cup	water	125 mL
2 tbsp	packed brown sugar	30 mL
1 tbsp	freshly squeezed lemon juice	15 mL
¼ tsp	ground cinnamon	1 mL

Yogurt Sauce

½ cup	lower-fat plain yogurt	125 mL
1 tbsp	packed brown sugar	15 mL
½ tsp	ground cinnamon	2 mL
½ tsp	vanilla extract	2 mL

1. Peel pears and cut in half lengthwise; scoop out core. Place cut side down in shallow baking dish. Sprinkle blueberries around pears.

2. Combine water, brown sugar, lemon juice and cinnamon; pour over pears. Bake, covered, in preheated oven for about 45 minutes or until pears are tender, basting occasionally with pan juices.

3. *Sauce:* In a small bowl, combine yogurt, brown sugar, cinnamon and vanilla. Serve pears with pan juices; spoon a dollop of yogurt sauce over cooked pear halves.

This recipe courtesy of Christine Cauch.

Nutrients
PER SERVING

Calories	167
Fat	1 g
Carbohydrate	40 g
Fiber	3 g
Protein	2 g

Fresh Berry Trifle

This trifle is lightened up with angel food cake, but it's still big on flavor.

Variation

Use instant vanilla or banana pudding instead of white chocolate.

- **Trifle bowl**

1	package (4-serving size) instant white chocolate pudding	1
1	10-inch (25 cm) angel food cake, torn into 1- to 2-inch (2.5 to 5 cm) cubes	1
½ cup	unsweetened orange juice	125 mL
5 cups	assorted berries (blueberries, raspberries, blackberries, strawberries)	1.25 L
1 cup	light whipped topping	250 mL

1. Prepare pudding according to package directions.
2. Place half the cake cubes in bottom of trifle bowl. Drizzle with half the orange juice. Spread half the pudding over cake and arrange one-third of the berries on top. Repeat layers of cake, juice, pudding and berries. Cover with whipped topping and top with the remaining berries.
3. Cover and refrigerate for at least 4 hours, until chilled, or for up to 12 hours.

This recipe courtesy of dietitian Brigitte Lamoureux.

Nutrients
PER SERVING

Calories	151
Fat	2 g
Carbohydrate	30 g
Fiber	3 g
Protein	4 g

Pumpkin Pie Tarts with Ground Almond Crust

These cute tarts give you all the flavor of pumpkin pie without the heavy pastry crust, and they make it easy to portion out Thanksgiving dessert!

Tip

You can make these tarts up to 2 days before you plan to serve them. Cover each ramekin with plastic wrap and refrigerate. Remove from refrigerator 30 minutes before serving.

Variation

Use ground pecans instead of almonds.

- **Preheat oven to 400°F (200°C)**
- **Eight ½-cup (125 mL) heatproof ramekins, greased**
- **2 baking sheets**

½ cup	ground almonds	125 mL
2	eggs, beaten	2
1¼ cups	canned pumpkin purée (not pie filling)	300 mL
½ cup	sweetened condensed milk	125 mL
1 tsp	ground cinnamon	5 mL
½ tsp	ground ginger	2 mL
¼ tsp	ground cloves	1 mL
¼ tsp	ground nutmeg	1 mL

1. Place 4 ramekins on each baking sheet. Divide ground almonds among prepared ramekins.

2. In a medium bowl, whisk together eggs, pumpkin, milk, cinnamon, ginger, cloves and nutmeg until well blended. Divide evenly among ramekins.

3. Bake in preheated oven for 10 minutes. Reduce oven temperature to 350°F (180°C) and bake for 12 to 15 minutes or until mostly set (the middle of the tarts should still jiggle slightly). Let cool completely in ramekins on a wire rack.

This recipe courtesy of dietitian Judy Campbell-Gordon.

Nutrients
PER SERVING

Calories	129
Fat	6 g
Carbohydrate	15 g
Fiber	2 g
Protein	5 g

Blueberry Semolina Cake

Talk about low-fat! This easy-to-make cake is a great way to serve fruit and still satisfy a sweet tooth. Serve warm for best results, and add fresh blueberries when serving.

Tips

If you reheat the cake a day later or after freezing, drizzle or brush an additional ¼ cup (60 mL) maple syrup over it to glaze.

Since blueberries have fragile skins, be gentle when folding them into any batter. Otherwise, the skins will break and the blueberries will leak their blue color into the cake.

Variation

Substitute your favorite fruit for blueberries.

- **Preheat oven to 325°F (160°C)**
- **8-inch (20 cm) square baking pan, lightly greased**

1½ cups	small semolina	375 mL
1 tsp	baking soda	5 mL
1 cup	lower-fat plain yogurt	250 mL
1 cup	fresh or frozen blueberries	250 mL
1 tsp	vanilla extract	5 mL
½ cup	pure maple syrup	125 mL

1. In a medium bowl, mix semolina and baking soda. Combine yogurt, blueberries and vanilla; stir into dry ingredients just until moistened. Do not overmix.

2. Spoon into prepared baking pan. Bake in preheated oven for 45 to 50 minutes or until tester inserted in center comes out clean. Remove cake from oven; pour syrup on top. Serve warm.

This recipe courtesy of chef Alain Mercier and dietitian Fabiola Masri.

Nutrients
PER SERVING

Calories	136
Fat	1 g
Carbohydrate	29 g
Fiber	1 g
Protein	4 g

Carrot Cake

This simple cake is a great way to add more vegetables to your diet.

Tip

Dust with icing sugar for a pretty presentation.

Variation

Combine grated apples with the carrots or use only apples for a change.

- Preheat oven to 350°F (180°C)
- 13- by 9-inch (33 by 23 cm) baking pan, lightly greased

¾ cup	all-purpose flour	175 mL
½ cup	whole wheat flour	125 mL
1¼ tsp	baking powder	6 mL
1¼ tsp	baking soda	6 mL
1 tsp	ground cinnamon	5 mL
½ tsp	salt	2 mL
3	eggs	3
½ cup	vegetable oil	125 mL
1 cup	lightly packed brown sugar	250 mL
2 tsp	vanilla extract	10 mL
2 cups	grated carrots	500 mL

1. In a small bowl, combine all-purpose flour, whole wheat flour, baking powder, baking soda, cinnamon and salt.

2. In a large bowl, beat eggs, oil, brown sugar and vanilla until well combined. Fold in dry ingredients. Stir in carrots. Pour into prepared pan.

3. Bake in preheated oven for 30 to 35 minutes or until a tester inserted in the center comes out clean. Let cool completely in pan on a wire rack. Cut cake into slices and lift servings out with a flat lifter.

This recipe courtesy of dietitian Shefali Raja.

Nutrients
PER SERVING

Calories	125
Fat	6 g
Carbohydrate	16 g
Fiber	1 g
Protein	2 g

Chocolate Zucchini Cake

This tasty chocolate cake has Mexican flair. Cocoa powder adds a satisfying chocolate flavor.

Tips

If you don't have self-rising flour, substitute 1 cup (250 mL) all-purpose flour and add 1½ tsp (7 mL) baking powder and ½ tsp (2 mL) salt.

If you prefer, use commercial liquid egg whites. You'll need about ¾ cup (175 mL) for this recipe.

- **Preheat oven to 350°F (180°C)**
- **8-inch (20 cm) square baking pan, lightly greased**

1 cup	self-rising flour	250 mL
⅓ cup	unsweetened cocoa powder	75 mL
1 tsp	baking soda	5 mL
1 tsp	ground cinnamon	5 mL
6	egg whites	6
1⅓ cups	firmly packed brown sugar	325 mL
1 cup	buttermilk	250 mL
2 tsp	vanilla extract	10 mL
¼ tsp	almond extract	1 mL
2 cups	shredded zucchini	500 mL
	Confectioners' (icing) sugar (optional)	

1. In a small bowl, sift flour, cocoa powder, baking soda and cinnamon.

2. In a large bowl, beat egg whites, brown sugar, buttermilk, vanilla and almond extract until well blended. Fold in flour mixture until evenly moistened. Stir in zucchini. Pour batter into prepared pan.

3. Bake in preheated oven for 30 to 40 minutes or until center of cake springs back when lightly pressed and a tester inserted in the center comes out clean. Let cool on a wire rack for 10 minutes before removing from pan. Turn out onto rack to cool completely. Just before serving, dust with confectioner's sugar, if desired.

This recipe courtesy of Eileen Campbell.

Nutrients PER SERVING	
Calories	154
Fat	1 g
Carbohydrate	35 g
Fiber	2 g
Protein	4 g

Applesauce Snack Cakes

**Makes
16 cupcakes**

Avoid excess sugar by knowing which foods are highest in added sugar. The most common sources are soft drinks, sports drinks and fruit drinks. You can also cut back on added sugar in recipes by one-quarter to one-third without sacrificing the end product.

Tips

Make your own applesauce when apples are plentiful and freeze in 2-cup (500 mL) portions.

For extra fiber, slide a wedge of unpeeled apple into the top of each snack cake before baking.

- **Preheat oven to 400°F (200°C)**
- **Two 8-cup muffin tins, greased or paper-lined**

½ cup	margarine	125 mL
1½ cups	granulated sugar	375 mL
2	eggs	2
1 tsp	vanilla extract	5 mL
2 cups	all-purpose flour	500 mL
1 tbsp	baking powder	15 mL
1 tsp	baking soda	5 mL
1½ tsp	ground cinnamon	7 mL
1 tsp	ground allspice	5 mL
½ tsp	ground cloves	2 mL
2 cups	unsweetened applesauce	500 mL

1. In a large bowl, cream margarine and sugar. Beat in eggs and vanilla until light and fluffy.

2. Sift together flour, baking powder, baking soda and spices. Add to creamed mixture alternately with applesauce, mixing well after each addition.

3. Spoon into prepared muffin cups, filling each about two-thirds full. Bake in preheated oven for about 20 minutes or until firm to the touch.

This recipe courtesy of Elaine Durst.

Nutrients
PER CUPCAKE

Calories	200
Fat	6 g
Carbohydrate	34 g
Fiber	1 g
Protein	2 g

Ginger Cookies

**Makes
30 cookies**

*A crisp, spicy cookie for
those who like the flavor
of gingerbread.*

- **Preheat oven to 350°F (180°C)**
- **Baking sheets, lightly greased or lined with parchment paper**

1¾ cups	all-purpose flour	425 mL
1½ tsp	baking powder	7 mL
1 tsp	ground ginger	5 mL
1 tsp	ground cinnamon	5 mL
½ tsp	baking soda	2 mL
½ tsp	salt	2 mL
¼ tsp	ground cloves	1 mL
1	egg	1
½ cup	granulated sugar	125 mL
½ cup	vegetable oil	125 mL
½ cup	light (fancy) molasses	125 mL

1. In a small bowl, combine flour, baking powder, ginger, cinnamon, baking soda, salt and cloves.

2. In a medium bowl, whisk egg, sugar, oil and molasses until blended. Fold in flour mixture until a moist dough forms.

3. Shape dough into balls, using about 1 tbsp (15 mL) dough per cookie, and place 2 inches (5 cm) apart on prepared baking sheets.

4. Bake in preheated oven for 10 to 12 minutes or until lightly browned and crisp. Let cool on baking sheets on a wire rack for 5 minutes, then remove to rack to cool completely.

This recipe courtesy of dietitian Phyllis Levesque.

Nutrients
PER COOKIE

Calories	91
Fat	4 g
Carbohydrate	13 g
Fiber	0 g
Protein	1 g

Rice Pudding

Rice pudding is a comfort-food favorite.

- **Four 1-cup (250 mL) ramekins**

1 cup	jasmine rice	250 mL
4 cups	unsweetened almond milk, divided	1 L
1	3-inch (7.5 cm) cinnamon stick	1
1/4 cup	pure maple syrup	60 mL
1 tsp	vanilla extract	5 mL
	Ground cinnamon	
	Ground nutmeg	

1. In a medium saucepan over medium-high heat, stir together rice, 3 cups (750 mL) of the almond milk and cinnamon stick and, stirring often, bring to a boil.

2. Reduce heat, cover and simmer for 15 to 20 minutes to partially cook rice. Stir in maple syrup, vanilla and remaining almond milk. Simmer, stirring and ensuring mixture doesn't become too dry, for 15 to 20 minutes or until most of the milk has been absorbed and rice is tender. Do not overcook.

3. Remove and discard cinnamon stick. Divide rice mixture evenly among ramekins. Sprinkle with cinnamon and nutmeg. Serve warm or cool.

Nutrients
PER SERVING

Calories	197
Fat	3 g
Carbohydrate	40 g
Fiber	2 g
Protein	3 g

Lemon-Lime Sorbet

*This is a fresh and tart
alternative to ice cream.*

- **Ice cream maker**

4 cups	lime-flavored club soda, divided	1 L
1 cup	granulated sugar	250 mL
1 cup	key lime preserves (without peel)	250 mL
	Juice of 2 lemons	
	Juice of 2 limes	

1. In a medium saucepan over low heat, stir together 1 cup (250 mL) of the club soda, sugar and preserves until sugar has dissolved and preserves have melted. Stir in lemon juice, lime juice and remaining soda. Pour into an airtight container and seal. Refrigerate for 2 to 3 hours or until thoroughly chilled.

2. Transfer to ice cream maker and process according to the manufacturer's instructions until mixture is the consistency of firm slush. Return to airtight container, seal and freeze for 1 hour or until mixture resembles sorbet.

Nutrients PER SERVING	
Calories	96
Fat	0 g
Carbohydrate	25 g
Fiber	0 g
Protein	0 g

Mango Mousse

How easy is it to create a versatile, refreshing dessert? Simply whirl two ingredients in a food processor, then top with fresh berries.

Tips

Mangos provide soluble fiber.

To make fruit parfaits, use tall parfait glasses. Layer in a half-serving of mousse, followed by a half-serving of berries. Repeat layers.

Serve in stemmed glasses for a buffet table.

• **Food processor**

1	bag (20 oz/600 g) frozen mango chunks, thawed and drained	1
½ cup	low-fat vanilla-flavored yogurt	125 mL
1 cup	sliced strawberries	250 mL
1 cup	blueberries	250 mL

1. In food processor, purée mango and yogurt for 1 minute or until smooth.

2. Divide mousse among serving bowls. Top with strawberries and blueberries and serve immediately, or cover and refrigerate for up to 12 hours, then top with berries before serving.

This recipe courtesy of dietitian Claude Gamache.

Nutrients
PER SERVING

Calories	80
Fat	1 g
Carbohydrate	19 g
Fiber	2 g
Protein	1 g

Contributing Authors

Dietitians of Canada
Cook Great Food
Recipes from this book are found on pages 146, 160, 165, 166, 181, 184, 187, 189, 191, 196, 198, 201, 205, 211, 218, 221, 225, 232, 242, 244, 247, 254, 260, 262, 265 and 268.

Dietitians of Canada
Simply Great Food
Recipes from this book are found on pages 147, 168, 171, 172, 174–76, 179, 182, 194, 210, 213, 219, 224, 228–30, 234–37, 241, 248, 253, 256, 266, 267 and 269.

Dr. Maitreyi Raman, Angela Sirounis and Jennifer Shrubsole
The Complete IBS Health & Diet Guide
Recipes from this book are found on pages 149, 151, 153, 162, 180, 199, 202, 203, 208, 212, 217, 220, 222, 251, 257–59, 270 and 271.

Mary Sue Waisman
Dietitians of Canada Cook!
Recipes from this book are found on pages 148, 150, 152, 154–59, 163, 164, 167, 170, 177, 178, 183, 186, 188, 190, 192, 193, 195, 200, 204, 206, 214, 216, 223, 226, 231, 238–40, 245, 246, 250, 252, 255, 263, 264 and 272.

Library and Archives Canada Cataloguing in Publication

Raman, Maitreyi
   Healing fatty liver disease : a complete health & diet guide, including 100 recipes / Maitreyi Raman, Angela Sirounis, Jennifer Shrubsole.

Includes index.
ISBN 978-0-7788-0437-6

1. Fatty liver—Popular works. 2. Fatty liver—Diet therapy—Popular works.
3. Fatty liver—Diet therapy—Recipes. 4. Cookbooks—
I. Sirounis, Angela II. Shrubsole, Jennifer III. Title.

RC848.F3R34 2013   616.3'62   C2012-907532-9

References

American Heart Association. Fish and omega-3 fatty acids. Available at: http://www.heart.org/HEARTORG/ GettingHealthy/NutritionCenter/HealthyDietGoals/ Fish-and-Omega-3-Fatty-Acids_UCM_303248_Article.jsp.

American Heart Association. Meet the fats. Available at: http://www.heart.org/HEARTORG/GettingHealthy/ FatsAndOils/Fats-Oils_UCM_001084_SubHomePage.jsp.

Barchetta I, Angelico F, Ben MD, et al. Strong association between non alcoholic fatty liver disease (NAFLD) and low 25(OH) vitamin D levels in an adult population with normal serum liver enzymes. *BMC Medicine* 2011;9:85. Available at: http://www.biomedcentral.com/1741-7015/9/85.

Dietitians of Canada. Food sources of chromium, molybdenum and fluoride. PEN: The Global Resource for Nutrition Practice.

Health Canada. Vitamin D and calcium: Updated dietary reference intakes. Available at: http://www.hc-sc.gc.ca/fn-an/ nutrition/vitamin/vita-d-eng.php.

Keating SE, Hackett DA, George J, et al. Exercise and non-alcoholic fatty liver disease: A systematic review and meta-analysis. *J Hepatol* 2012;57(1):157–66.

Parnell JA, Raman M, Rioux KP, et al. The potential role of prebiotic fibre for treatment and management of non-alcoholic fatty liver disease and associated obesity and insulin resistance. *Liver Int* 2012 May;32(5):701–11.

Parrish CR. Nutritional recommendations for patients with non-alcoholic fatty liver disease: An evidence based review. *Practical Gastroenterology* 2010 Feb;82:8–16.

Index

More Great Books
from Robert Rose

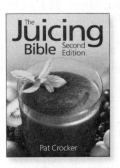

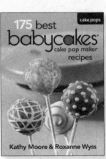

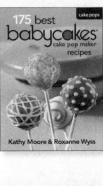

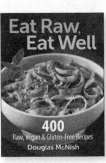

Bestsellers

- The Juicing Bible, Second Edition
  by Pat Crocker
- 175 Best Babycakes™ Cupcake Maker Recipes
  by Kathy Moore and Roxanne Wyss
- 175 Best Babycakes™ Cake Pop Maker Recipes
  by Kathy Moore and Roxanne Wyss
- Eat Raw, Eat Well
  by Douglas McNish
- Best of Bridge Slow Cooker Cookbook
  by Best of Bridge and Sally Vaughan-Johnston
- The Food Substitutions Bible, Second Edition
  by David Joachim
- Zwilling J.A. Henckels Complete Book of Knife Skills
  by Jeffrey Elliot and James P. DeWan

Appliance Bestsellers

- 225 Best Pressure Cooker Recipes
  by Cinda Chavich
- 200 Best Panini Recipes
  by Tiffany Collins
- 125 Best Indoor Grill Recipes
  by Ilana Simon
- The Convection Oven Bible
  by Linda Stephen
- The Fondue Bible
  by Ilana Simon

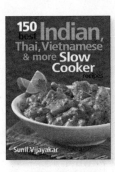

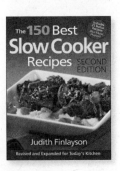

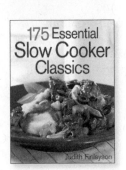

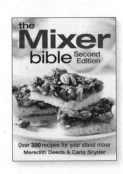

- 150 Best Indian, Thai, Vietnamese & More Slow Cooker Recipes
  by Sunil Vijayakar
- The 150 Best Slow Cooker Recipes, Second Edition
  by Judith Finlayson
- The Vegetarian Slow Cooker
  by Judith Finlayson
- 175 Essential Slow Cooker Classics
  by Judith Finlayson
- The Healthy Slow Cooker
  by Judith Finlayson
- Slow Cooker Winners
  by Donna-Marie Pye
- Canada's Slow Cooker Winners
  by Donna-Marie Pye
- 300 Best Rice Cooker Recipes
  by Katie Chin
- 650 Best Food Processor Recipes
  by George Geary and Judith Finlayson
- The Mixer Bible, Second Edition
  by Meredith Deeds and Carla Snyder
- 300 Best Bread Machine Recipes
  by Donna Washburn and Heather Butt
- 300 Best Canadian Bread Machine Recipes
  by Donna Washburn and Heather Butt

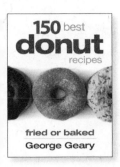

Baking Bestsellers

- 150 Best Cupcake Recipes
  by Julie Hasson
- Piece of Cake!
  by Camilla V. Saulsbury
- 400 Sensational Cookies
  by Linda J. Amendt
- Complete Cake Mix Magic
  by Jill Snider
- 150 Best Donut Recipes
  by George Geary
- 750 Best Muffin Recipes
  by Camilla V. Saulsbury
- 200 Fast & Easy Artisan Breads
  by Judith Fertig

Healthy Cooking Bestsellers

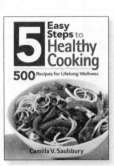

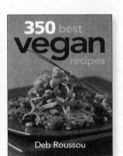

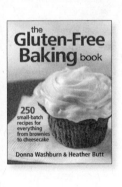

- Canada's Diabetes Meals for Good Health, Second Edition
  by Karen Graham
- Diabetes Meals for Good Health, Second Edition
  by Karen Graham
- 5 Easy Steps to Healthy Cooking
  by Camilla V. Saulsbury
- 350 Best Vegan Recipes
  by Deb Roussou
- The Vegan Cook's Bible
  by Pat Crocker
- The Gluten-Free Baking Book
  by Donna Washburn and Heather Butt
- Complete Gluten-Free Cookbook
  by Donna Washburn and Heather Butt

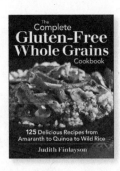

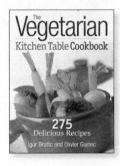

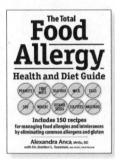

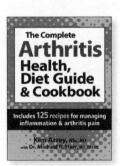

- 250 Gluten-Free Favorites
  by Donna Washburn and Heather Butt
- Complete Gluten-Free Diet & Nutrition Guide
  by Alexandra Anca and Theresa Santandrea-Cull
- The Complete Gluten-Free Whole Grains Cookbook
  by Judith Finlayson
- The Vegetarian Kitchen Table Cookbook
  by Igor Brotto and Olivier Guiriec

Health Bestsellers

- The Total Food Allergy Health and Diet Guide
  by Alexandra Anca with Dr. Gordon L. Sussman
- The Complete Arthritis Health, Diet Guide & Cookbook
  by Kim Arrey with Dr. Michael R. Starr
- The Essential Cancer Treatment Nutrition Guide & Cookbook
  by Jean LaMantia with Dr. Neil Berinstein
- The Complete Weight-Loss Surgery Guide & Diet Program
  by Sue Ekserci with Dr. Laz Klein
- The PCOS Health & Nutrition Guide
  by Dr. Jillian Stansbury with Dr. Sheila Mitchell

By the same authors

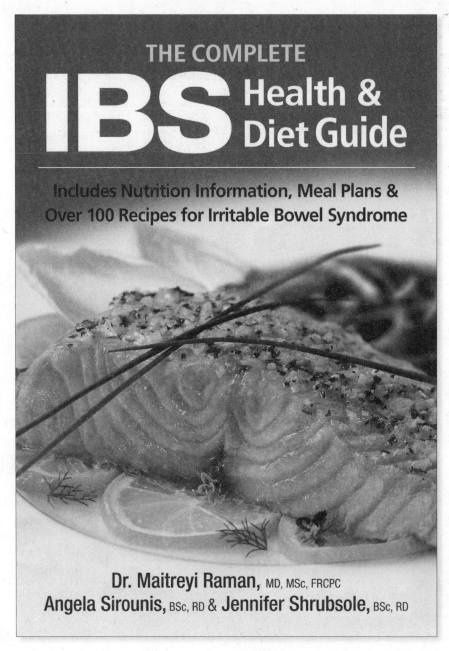

THE COMPLETE

IBS Health & Diet Guide

Includes Nutrition Information, Meal Plans & Over 100 Recipes for Irritable Bowel Syndrome

Dr. Maitreyi Raman, MD, MSc, FRCPC
Angela Sirounis, BSc, RD & **Jennifer Shrubsole,** BSc, RD

ISBN 978-0-7788-0263-1